Self-Inquiry

–

Dawn of the Witness
and
The End of Suffering

Yogani

D1471435

From The AYP Enlightenment Series

AYP Publishing

For ordering information go to:

www.advancedyogapractices.com

Library of Congress Control Number: 2007924701

Published simultaneously in:

Nashville, Tennessee, U.S.A.
and
London, England, U.K.

This title is also available in eBook format – ISBN 978-0-9800522-2-0
(For Adobe Reader)

ISBN 978-0-9800522-0-6 (Paperback)

"You will know the truth,
and the truth will set you free."

John 8:32

Introduction

With *Deep Meditation* and the rise of abiding inner silence (the witness), we find ourselves with an increasing ability to observe our thoughts as objects. This volume on *Self-Inquiry* provides practical approaches for making use of our inner witness in daily activity and relationships, resulting in increased inner stability and happiness amidst the ups and downs of life. The prudent use of self-inquiry also enables us to realize the ultimate truth of existence – the *Oneness* we are and the *Unity* of all that exists.

It is hoped that this sharing will help bring clarity to the often misunderstood field of self-inquiry by revealing the relationship between our undifferentiated consciousness (subject/witness) and our thoughts, feelings and perceptions of the material world (objects). The philosophical schools expounding the so-called *dual* and *non-dual* views of existence have sometimes been at odds, even though they have been describing the same thing.

When our nervous system is systematically cultivated in ways that bring deep purification and opening, then we will be able to directly perceive the reality of *Self* and the true nature of the world, and describe it first-hand. The relevance of our own experience will surpass the philosophies that have informed us in the past, and we will know the truth.

The Advanced Yoga Practices Enlightenment Series is an endeavor to present the most effective methods of spiritual practice in a series of easy-to-read books that anyone can use to gain practical results immediately and over the long term. For centuries, many of these powerful practices have been shrouded in secrecy, mainly in an effort to preserve them. Now we find ourselves in the *information age*, and able to preserve knowledge for present and future generations like never before. The question remains: "How far can we go in effectively transmitting spiritual methods in writing?"

Since its beginnings in 2003, the writings of *Advanced Yoga Practices* have been an experiment to see just how much can be conveyed, with much more detail included on practices than in the spiritual writings of the past. Can books provide us the specific means necessary to tread the path to enlightenment, or do we have to surrender at the feet of a *guru* to find our salvation? Well, clearly we must surrender to something, even if it is to our own innate potential to live a freer and happier life. If we are able to do that, and maintain regular practice, then books like this one can come alive and instruct us in the ways of human spiritual transformation. If the reader is ready and the book is worthy, amazing things can happen.

While one person's name is given as the author of this book, it is actually a distillation of the efforts of thousands of practitioners over thousands of years. This is one person's attempt to simplify and make practical the spiritual methods that many have demonstrated throughout history. All who have gone before have my deepest gratitude, as do the many I am privileged to be in touch with in the present who continue to practice with dedication and good results.

I hope you will find this book to be a useful resource as you travel along your chosen path.

Practice wisely, and enjoy!

Table of Contents

Chapter 1 – On the Trail of Truth

We would all like to know *the truth* of our existence on this earth. Throughout our life we may seek it by asking questions like,

"*Who am I?*"

"*What am I doing here?*"

"*Who or what is God?*"

"*What is the real nature of things?*"

"*Is what I am experiencing right now really true?*"

And so on...

If we ask our questions with feeling and persistence, if we continue to *inquire*, the answers will come to us sooner or later. How we go about it will determine our rate of progress, and the degree of ease or difficulty we may experience on the road to knowledge. Therefore, a methodology with predictable results can bring some important benefits. We will attempt to deliver a reliable approach to the field of self-inquiry here. It is a novel idea, because the traditional approaches to self-inquiry are often accompanied by much uncertainty, for reasons that will become clear as we move along. Is such uncertainty necessary? Not really. It is only a matter of gaining some education and understanding of the dynamics of human spiritual transformation. With some practical perspective, the journey can be made without pulling the hinges off the divine doorway of our nervous system.

It is a paradox that formal structured approaches to self-inquiry can lead to uncertainty and limited results. We will reveal why this is so. Here, we will take a less structured approach, and not offer a *cookbook* for self-inquiry. There are plenty of these available already. Instead, we will look at underlying principles, and how we can apply these principles in concert with continuing spiritual progress resulting from a balanced *integration* of effective yoga practices.

Through endless inquiry and experimentation over the centuries, humankind has made much progress in determining the truth about our world, and beyond, to the point where applied science has harnessed many principles in nature for our betterment. Some may argue whether all of this progress has been for the better. Nevertheless, the steady expansion of applied knowledge marches on, and we are obliged to make the best of it. Such a progressive approach for the application of steadily accumulating knowledge can also be used in the development and implementation of practical spiritual methods. It is time for that.

In spite of our increasing mastery of the material laws of nature and this small planet we live on, we have done little so far to realize the ultimate truth of who we are and what we are doing here, let alone make much practical use of that elusive knowledge. Because of this we continue to suffer at the hands of our perceived mortality.

If finding the truth were simply a matter of developing an intellectual understanding, it would be easy – as easy as taking a high school class in physics, including an introduction to the principles of quantum mechanics. With that, we will know that all we see and do in life is playing out in a vast realm of *absolute emptiness*, with innumerable bits of interacting energy creating the appearance and substance of everything we consider to be our real world.

So, how *real* is our world, if all we are seeing, hearing and touching is nothing but energy interacting with itself in vast emptiness? This is a question that cannot be avoided when considering the ultimate consequences of quantum mechanics. Why is there an apparent inconsistency between what physics tells us and the physical world we perceive around us? And how does this inconsistency affect the quality of our life? Can knowing the truth about this alleviate our suffering, as wise people both ancient and modern have promised?

We can find out for ourselves through direct experience.

It is a matter of perception. To experience and know more, our perception must be refined. While we cannot perceive radio waves with our normal senses, we have developed the technology to perceive them, and use them for great benefit. Modern technology has opened many doors for us in this way.

Interestingly, the ancient science of *Yoga* goes quite a lot further than modern science has so far in dealing with the unseen realm of absolute emptiness we are purported to be made of and living in. While modern science relies on devices enabling us to perceive and utilize principles in nature that we cannot see, the field of yoga relies on the human nervous system to do the same thing, and with remarkable results.

While utilizing our own nervous system as the primary instrument for discerning and applying the ultimate truth of life may seem like a new idea, there have been small groups of people doing it for thousands of years. It has been a fragile affair, with many disruptions and distortions coming from the forces of chaos that have been running roughshod over humanity for many centuries. The great religions of the world have spun off and grown from these small groups of spiritual innovators, inevitably mixing the truth in with politics and the long-running struggle of humanity to survive and thrive.

Now we find ourselves in the *information age*, where knowledge can be more easily distilled, preserved and shared, and it is more difficult for the forces of chaos to have their way. In this way, modern information technology has come to lend a hand to the ancient science of spirit.

Due to the rapid rise of knowledge, we have arrived at a turning point, a point where many people around the world can deepen their inquiry about the nature of things, shifting the perspective from being outside ourselves to include a more penetrating inquiry from the point of view of what is inside us – our radiant inner *Self*.

This has been made possible by the rise of knowledge about integrated spiritual practices in the modern world, with the principles and methods of practical *self-inquiry* being part of that.

Self-Inquiry – The Yoga of Knowledge

Self-inquiry is not new. It has been part of yoga and other systems of spiritual practice for centuries. It has been called *jnana yoga*, meaning "union through knowledge." Jnana means *knowledge*, and yoga means *union* of the inner and outer aspects of life. Self-inquiry has also been called the *path of discrimination* and the *path of the intellect*. Knowledge of what? Discrimination of what? Intellectual knowledge of what? These are fair questions, and we will attempt to answer them in this book. Jnana also means *wisdom*, which points to a deeper level of knowing, a spiritual knowing, which is the end game of self-inquiry, and all of yoga.

Before we delve into the particulars of self-inquiry and additional yoga practices upon which its success depends, let's look at the relationship of philosophy and experience, which can help form a framework and basis for a practical approach to self-inquiry.

Roles of Philosophy and Experience

As we begin to think about the true nature of things, it is helpful to have a foundation in the form of an idea or structure. Quantum physics was mentioned for this reason, offering the modern scientific model of emptiness underlying our physical universe. The ancient philosophical traditions of the East concur with this view, with an additional component added – the presence of *consciousness* in absolute emptiness and emerging from it. While it may not be possible to verify that the emptiness underlying everything is conscious, we can certainly verify that what manifests from emptiness is conscious, because we are conscious.

Ancient eastern philosophy, and some western philosophies also, hold emptiness to the great *Self* of all, and that all individual selves are but rays emanating from the *One Great Self*, much the way waves dance upon the surface of the ocean, only to dissolve and reappear on the surface of the ocean again and again. The waves are ever-changing expressions of the great ocean they dance upon.

Whether the great ocean of emptiness beyond the manifested universe is conscious can be debated. But there can be little debate about whether human beings are conscious. It is this singular fact that underlies the entire field of self-inquiry.

There is a vast theoretical body of knowledge, which can be found in the amply documented philosophies of both the East and the West, plus the experiential component of consciousness which can be found in every human being. Put these two together, and you have the beginnings of self-inquiry.

It is really quite simple. If we can come to know that we are, in fact, the ocean before, during and after we are the wave, then the inquiry is done. Enlightenment is ours. Philosophically, that is called the *end of knowledge*. In the East, it is called *Vedanta – the end of the Veda*.

But, experientially, it is not so simple. Something more is needed, which is often overlooked by those who hold an uncompromising view of human enlightenment. If our experience does not fulfill the philosophy, or even what another may claim as their experience, then the inquiry is not complete. While purists may hold that only emptiness exists, it is up to each of us to verify the truth for ourselves. It is for this that the methods of self-inquiry are given.

But it turns out that self-inquiry is very much a moving target, depending on the person who is doing it. Just as certain ideas will resonate with some people and not others, the methods of self-inquiry may resonate with some practitioners and not with others. The reason for this variation is due to the inner condition of each individual nervous system. The degree of inner purification and opening deep inside has a direct bearing on the degree of consciousness that is available in the person for gaining knowledge of the nature of existence, at least insofar as knowledge can be gained through direct experience within the individual.

The key factor in this is the presence of what we call inner silence, also called pure bliss consciousness, the *Self*, or the *witness*. It is called the witness because stillness in our awareness is our ground state and, once established, is capable of experiencing all thoughts, perceptions and emotions as objects outside its own unmoving awareness.

The presence of the witness changes the complexion and effectiveness of all self-inquiry methods dramatically, and our perception of every day living also. What had been a moving target becomes steady, and the very knowledge we have been seeking is what we become. We were *That* all along, and the witness is *That*. There is the old saying that, what we are seeking is what is doing the seeking. Our inner awareness in the form of the witness is both the goal and the means for attaining it.

The witness can be cultivated in human beings by engaging in self-inquiry. This is its purpose. However, it is very difficult to do it using self-inquiry as the sole means. Ask anyone who has tried without using any other supporting practices.

A much more effective way to cultivate the witness is with daily *deep meditation*. Once this kind of cultivation is occurring on an ongoing basis, then self-inquiry will have the ability to gain some real traction in our lives, and add far-reaching additional benefits that could not be realized with either deep meditation or self-inquiry alone. When we say "traction," we mean the formation of an intimate *relationship* between our native consciousness and the objects of this world, including our thoughts, feelings and perceptions of the external environment. Our abiding inner witness, combined with self-inquiry, can lead us steadily toward a condition of *Oneness*, beyond the ups and downs of life, even as we are fully engaged and going about our business each day. In this condition, there is not grasping or hanging on.

So, if we are looking for real self-inquiry, we should look beyond the dictums of rigid philosophical systems to the inner workings of our own nervous system. If we do that, we will go beyond ideas to the experience itself. Then the wave will know itself to be the ocean, even as it continues as a wave.

Philosophy is therefore a stepping stone to the greatest knowledge, which is direct knowledge of our *Self*.

The Importance of Practice

There are those who say that practice is not necessary to reach enlightenment. Indeed, the unconditioned state of pure bliss consciousness is beyond all practice. So they are right in saying that the end state is beyond all practice, and even beyond all experience. When the fluctuations of the mind have been transcended, only the absolute remains. To be in this condition, nothing must be done, and nothing is, at least from the point of view of someone who is in this state on an ongoing basis. But what about everyone else?

The advice not to practice is an extremist view that leads many into confusion, particularly those who have responsibilities in the world. Such advice may be interpreted to mean going on with life as it has always been (having learned what?), or rejecting life completely in favor of *doing nothing*. Either way, there will be a problem.

So, while philosophically the argument not to practice, or do nothing, has appeal, on the practical level it has little relationship to what most people are involved with in daily life – living and doing. And neither is the advice to not practice particularly helpful for people who are contemplative in their nature, as it will often be interpreted to mean sitting around all day doing nothing.

The question is not so much about whether practice is necessary or not. Practice is not the enemy. Effective practice is about changing the point of view of the practitioner (you and me) in relation to the objects of our experience. Consciousness as it manifests through us has a strong tendency to identify with everything it experiences, mistaking itself to be the objects it is observing. This includes the very thoughts and feelings we are having right now.

Once identified with external phenomena, our awareness will say, "I am these thoughts and feelings. I am this body. This is my family, my nation and my world."

Once this occurs, we are on the roller coaster of life – the *wheel of birth and death*, as the philosophers say. It is very much a dream we create for ourselves.

Those who see through the illusion we have built up within and around ourselves will say, "Just stop identifying with all this. Do nothing. Let it all go!"

There is a certain amount of determination a teacher may have in wanting to wake people up to *what is*. Lacking more practical means, a teacher may resort to radical advice, which will not be able to be implemented by most people with any degree of reliability.

There are several problems with this radical approach. First, doing nothing is doing something. On the level of the mind, the act of letting go is a doing, so it will be a contrary experience for many people. And it is not so easy anyway for most people who are living regular lives. Attempting to take such a radical view with the mind can actually be very destructive to the motivation of the person and seriously disrupt effectiveness in daily life.

So perhaps the conclusion will be to go off to a remote cave where letting go and doing nothing might be more doable. But, alas, there is a problem with this

*The witness is inner Silence —
The practice is achieve inner silence*

too. Our mind goes with us to the cave, and all that we have been identified with goes with us also. We take ourselves wherever we go.

The *don't practice* guru will tell us to be vigilant in doing nothing. We should *practice* this in our every waking moment!

It is pretty silly, isn't it? Building a mountain of intention and mental strategies, all for the purpose of doing nothing. The mind can never figure itself out. Only by transcending the mind can we know what the mind and everything else really is.

Once we have come to the recognition that doing nothing is actually doing something, we can begin to take a more practical approach, by doing something that actually can work. And that something is engaging in methods that can gradually dissolve the identification of our awareness with the objects of perception. As this identification and the dream we have been in begin to dissolve, the experience will be the rise of inner silence, our consciousness without the encumbrance of identification with the objects of perception, including our own thoughts. This unencumbered awareness, we call the *witness*.

The witness is not a condition we conjure up in the mind. It cannot be manufactured by the mind. It is a real and permanent presence of our awareness devoid of attachment to the experiences of temporal life. The witness is beyond the mind. Cultivating the witness is the object of self-inquiry, and of all yoga. Later on, we will learn how the witness also becomes dynamic, illuminating all objects we perceive, from within. Then we are able to do everything without doing anything. But it takes some particular kinds of doing to cultivate this condition of non-doing. This is the outcome of combining a full range of yoga practices.

Real & permanent PRESENCE
AWARENESS
the end of suffering

While there is a strong tendency for teachers and practitioners to cling to a singular methodology for producing spiritual progress, this is not the most effective approach. It doesn't matter what method is touted as *the way*. There simply is not a single way that will carry everyone through to the realization we all seek.

The methods of yoga are not mutually exclusive. They are mutually integrative. Bypassing the full range of yoga methods that are available in favor of a fixation on a single method is a risky proposition at best. Maybe there will be some results, and maybe there won't. It will depend more on the initial condition of the practitioner than on the method itself. Of course, the initial condition of the practitioner will always determine the initial results. In fact, we could say that those who tend to oversimplify the task of revealing the truth within all of us were naturals from the beginning, needing very little in the way of practice, and what they offer is suitable only for those who are nearly enlightened already also.

And what about the rest of us?

We want more than philosophical platitudes that might tickle a sense of the infinite residing within us. We want to realize it. For this, we have an array of practices that can be integrated in a highly complementary way. Self-inquiry is one of these practices, and it comes into play in a variety of ways in relation to our over all strategy of daily yoga practices.

Let's delve deeper.

Chapter 2 – An Approach to Self-Inquiry

While we may often hear that enlightenment is an absolute condition which can be realized immediately by using absolute measures, this is fiction for the vast majority of people. It is an attractive proposition for the mind. We could even say that it is intellectually and emotionally seductive. But it is fiction all the same. Taking such thinking too seriously may lead us to extremist approaches that can delay our spiritual progress rather than enhance it.

There is a middle way.

As soon as we come to the realization that enlightenment is a *journey* rather than an instant event, we will open to the possibilities, and many doors will begin to open. If we remain open, we will find that an integration of methods can bring us to realize what we have been seeking, and with far less effort. Ironically, the multifold path is the path of least doing, and certainly the one of least angst.

Could it be that simple?

The AYP approach to self-inquiry is to integrate it naturally into our life as part of our over all routine of practices. In part, self-inquiry is what we have the option to do as we go about our normal every day life, between our twice-daily sittings of structured practices. Self-inquiry of this kind is less structured and highly individual. It may draw on different teachings at different times. However, there are several levels of application in self-inquiry which are essential to understand, mainly so we can stay in synchronization with our own spiritual progress. It is important to understand where we are in relation to our practice, and pace our practice to accommodate the changes that are occurring within us. This applies to self-inquiry as much as with any other practice we are utilizing. So we will be systematic in our approach here, but not issuing *cookbook* instructions for self-inquiry. Our practice will be determined by our own inner inclinations and the application of sound principles. It is the most progressive and safe approach to spiritual development, assuming we are working with the underlying principles of human spiritual transformation and integrating time-tested techniques.

We will be doing many things in order to be doing nothing in the stillness of our inner awareness.

The primary aim of self-inquiry is to remain established in the unconditioned inner silence that resides within all of us – the experiencer, the witness to all thoughts, feelings and perceptions of the body and external phenomena.

Self-inquiry seeks to dissolve the identification of awareness with all of these perceptions. The traditional wisdom holds that the abiding presence of the witness (undifferentiated consciousness) will be the *effect* of self-inquiry. It can be, and this is the aim of all who pursue self-inquiry as a stand-alone path. All of the various strategies (*mental algorithms*) of self-inquiry are for realizing *That*.

However, it is also true that the presence of the witness is the *cause* of self-inquiry. When the witness is present, a natural inclination toward self-inquiry becomes self-evident, for then the innate condition of the practitioner *as the witness* becomes the answer to every inquiry – the eternal stillness that does nothing even as life carries on in all of its diversity. Once the witness is present, self-inquiry becomes more or less automatic. The witness is both the fuel and the destination of self-inquiry.

In the AYP approach, we seek to cultivate the witness <u>first</u> by the most effective means at our disposal.

We begin by establishing a practice of daily deep meditation. In doing so, we insure the fruition of all we undertake in self-inquiry, and our permanent realization of the truth.

Deep Meditation and the Inner Witness

Deep meditation is a specific practice that is designed to cultivate inner silence, which is the witness, regarded to be a prerequisite for self-inquiry in the AYP approach. Deep meditation is a very simple practice, and is very powerful. So powerful that it only needs to be practiced for 15-20 minutes twice daily. That is more than enough to set us on the road of cultivating the witness, and self-inquiry grows naturally out of that.

This style of meditation involves the use of a *mantra*, and repeatedly refining it to stillness with a specific procedure. The mantra used is *I AM*, and the procedure involves mental repetition of the mantra without regard to meaning. Deep meditation is not an inquiry into the meaning of *I AM*. It is systematically transcending the vibration of *I AM* in the mind to stillness. In this way, stillness is cultivated in the mind, not only during deep meditation, but, more importantly, during the time we are not meditating in our daily activities. Then inner silence comes to be known as a witnessing quality in our life, which opens up the possibility for more effective self-inquiry. When we have inner silence, self-inquiry is the natural result, because we will come to know our thoughts and feelings to be objects of perception, rather than who we are. It becomes evident that we are the witness, and all the rest can be released or engaged in without the bondage of the identification of awareness with the experiences of life.

Becoming the witness also leads to the end of suffering, for suffering ceases when awareness is no longer identified with pain. Pain will still be there as before, along with all the rest of life's experiences, but suffering will not be there. Suffering is the identification of the mind with pain, discomfort and the failure of desires to be fulfilled. When we have become the witness, we will still experience all of these things on the surface, but will not suffer within ourselves. Self-inquiry has a key role to play in completing the realization that the witness, who we are, does not suffer. Indeed, self-inquiry is an ideal practice for completing the journey of our witness-Self becoming free of the last traces of the identification of our awareness with the temporal aspects of life.

Does this mean we leave life, cease to be engaged or interested in what is going on around us? No, it does not mean that. It is quite to the contrary. The cultivation of inner silence via deep meditation enhances positive qualities within us – the flowering of compassion, love, and the energy to engage in the world in evolutionary ways. This may seem in contrast to the classical view of self-inquiry, which may exhort us to drop all attachments in the world. With the rise of the witness, that is in fact what happens. We cease to be identified with the goings on in time and space, while at the same time we overflow with outpouring love in the very realm we have transcended. We can let go of the world even as we are illuminating it naturally from within. Our actions will tell the tale, for we will be doing much more for others, even as we are doing less inside. This is the power of the witness when cultivated into full presence within the individual.

Inner silence is at the heart of all of yoga, and at the heart of all systems of spiritual knowledge and unfoldment. Without inner silence, there would be no systems of spiritual development. Inner silence is the spirit within us and all things.

All spiritual paths are about revealing our *"I,"* and becoming it in its native unconditioned state. All spiritual paths are for answering the question *"Who am I?"* and consciously becoming *That.* Our nervous system has the ability to reveal that reality within us, and more. This is why we call the human nervous system the doorway to the infinite.

With direct experience through deep meditation, self-inquiry, and other integrated practices, we can go from the philosophy/theory of inner silence to the reality of it. The leap from theory to reality is found in the ways that our nervous system manifests different forms of awareness. The witness alive in us is known to be that ever-awake sense of *"I"* during waking, dreaming and deep sleep stages of awareness. Inner silence is a state distinctly different from these other three. In deep meditation, it is blissful awareness without any objects. Once cultivated as distinct, the witness will be there underlying all objects also – our thoughts, feelings, and external experiences.

The difference between inner silence and the temporal states of waking, dreaming and deep sleep states of consciousness is that inner silence is unchanging and can be cultivated in the nervous system as an unending presence superimposed under, in, and through the other three states of consciousness.

With daily deep meditation, inner silence begins as some inner peace and an awareness of a silent quality coexisting with and within the objects of our perception in daily living. This happens with external observations through the senses, and with our thoughts and feelings. We see them as the objects that they are, occurring external to our unconditioned inner silent awareness. With a continuation of daily deep meditation and the integration of additional practices that are available, inner silence grows and becomes the movie screen upon which all our experiences are projected. We become the movie screen – the infinite movie screen of life. It is what we are. It is our essential nature.

Inner silence is the space between our thoughts. It is the gap we sometimes experience as we pass from one thought to another, and from one state of consciousness to another. When the music stops for an instant, we are left with inner silence, our true *Self.*

Keep in mind that inner silence is not on the level of the curious mind or the intellect. It is beyond all thinking and philosophy. In that sense the call to do nothing is valid. In order to do that we must do something.

Daily practices are for purifying and opening our nervous system – a dramatic expansion of the functioning of our neurobiology, leading to true knowledge of what is. So, cultivating inner silence directly through daily deep meditation has far-reaching implications in our approach to self-inquiry, and in the quality of our life – a life that can be lived in fulfillment, without suffering.

Self-Inquiry – From Inspiration to Realization

Next to devotion, which is the cornerstone of all the spiritual traditions of the world, self-inquiry is the most common spiritual technique on the earth. In fact, it isn't even considered a spiritual technique by many who engage in it. It is simply an ongoing inquiry for truth.

As little children it is likely we have asked, "*Who am I?*" and "*Why am I here?*" The way in which we have answered these questions in the past has determined to a large degree what we have done with our lives up until now. And if we have not been too hardened by life, we are likely to still be asking these questions. We are wired for it. We simply must know the truth about life. It is an endless search for purpose and meaning.

Perhaps at some point we read or heard that life is unbounded and that human beings can experience this unbounded nature of life, and become *That*. Somehow it rang true, and we were inspired. Perhaps we have been inspired ever since.

It is from there that we began our quest for knowledge in earnest, only to find that the mind alone, while very good for entertaining ideas, even one so grand as *enlightenment*, will leave us either stuck in frustration or lost in a labyrinth of endless streams of thought. Even the thought of letting go can create more mental structure and inertia.

The more we think about it, the more frustrating it can become. The mind just isn't the place to solve the riddle of enlightenment. The key is to go beyond the mind. We don't have to kill our mind or our thoughts to do this. We just need to find our center in the witness, which is beyond the mind, and easily favor that. Then the mind becomes our friend again. The mind makes a

DIS-IDENTIFY WITH the Mind.

Self-hypnosis suggestion.

poor master, but a very good servant. Our goal is not to get rid of the mind or thinking. The goal is to dissolve the identification of our mind as our self, our ego, to wake up from the dream that we have been living in. It is not the destruction of the ego or the mind. Only a shift to become identified as the great blank screen behind the grand movie of our life – the witness.

So, it is very important what we do with the inspiration that our initial self-inquiry may bring us. If we use the inspiration to propel us into sound methods for transcending the mind to stillness, then we will find the possibility to move from inspiration to transformation.

The idealist touting a philosophical approach will say that there is no transformation to be had, for everything is as it should be right now. We only must realize it in the now. But that realization is a transformation also, and it cannot occur until our perception is opened to a level where we can see *what is*. Without the witness, it will not happen.

It is possible to spend many years in self-inquiry, pondering the truth behind things and studying the words of *those who know* over and over again. Such writings are plentiful, easily accessed these days, and can be very inspiring. Yet, no matter how many times we read the words, or engage in the logic of particular modes of self-inquiry, we may feel quite distant from what the words and ideas are attempting to convey. The reason is because we can only know within ourselves, and for that, the perception of our own inner silence as our *Self* must be opened. We need the witness.

Then, when we read the words of the wise, they will resonate more each time. It will not be the words that change us. It will be we who have changed, and we will

Self hypnosis 2 access the witness.

see more truth in all expressions of knowledge as we continue to open to our native awareness inside.

Self-inquiry itself is not a very effective way to cultivate the witness. It is the underlying principle of meditation that cultivates the witness – always. To the extent self-inquiry can aid us in dissolving the objects of the mind, it will cultivate the witness. In doing so, it will be utilizing the principle of meditation – gradually dissolving the identification of our awareness with objects to become increasingly identified with the subject, which is the witness. Self-inquiry is not necessarily the most efficient kind of meditation, but it can be a kind of meditation all the same.

The important thing about our early days of self-inquiry, and our budding desire for truth, is that we transform the inspiration gained into useful measures that will unfold the witness within us. If we do that, then we will find ourselves coming back to self-inquiry later on with much more clarity than we had in the beginning. So the approach that is suggested here is to inquire, be inspired, unfold the witness in daily deep meditation, and then inquire some more when the urge arises naturally from within us, as it surely will. This is an approach that is self-sustaining and will lead to much progress, peace and joy in life.

It is the journey from inspiration to realization, and what we do in-between will make all the difference.

Thy will B Done –
Self awareness – mindfullness

Relational and Non-Relational Self-Inquiry

In its purest form, self-inquiry takes the position that nothing exists. There is only *I AM*. In fact, in pure self-inquiry, there is no *"I,"* for *"I"* must utilize a vehicle of expression. And *AM* does not exist either. The self-awareness of *AM* cannot be verified, except as a sense of *being* described after the fact. The description of the *AM* is only that, a description. The same can be said of the witness, even if we are self-identified with it at all times. The witness is awareness independent of all objects. Yet, the witness does coexist with objects, as anyone who engages in daily deep meditation for a while knows. So we can try and describe it, even though it is who we are beyond all descriptions. It is a riddle.

The coexistence of the witness with objects is not generally accepted by those engaged in the most uncompromising forms of self-inquiry, even as they engage with objects and walk about doing daily activities ranging from the mundane to the complex. Their assertion is that there are no objects. In uncompromising approaches to self-inquiry, we are instructed to let life go and reside in *That* which is behind the illusion. We are told, "Be the blank screen behind the movie."

It is all well and good. It is the truth. We are *That* and all objects are projections within *That*. However, this kind of thinking will only be *thinking* if there is no abiding witness present while such concepts are being entertained. And therein lies the problem, a flaw in the impeccable logic of pure uncompromising self-inquiry.

The premise is that if one engages in this kind of thinking for long enough, then eventually the letting go that results will lead to *realization*, and the cognition of

That which is beyond the play occurring in time and space, which is presumed to have no reality whatsoever. This "realization" can be instant. So it is said.

There is an inconsistency in this approach. Not for everyone, but for a large percentage of the population. The problem is that for those who are yet to cultivate abiding inner silence (the witness) this kind of self-inquiry will be largely intellectual. That which is being sought in letting go is a thought object in the mind also. So it is thoughts about thoughts. The mind playing with the mind. It can go on for a very long time.

This kind of self-inquiry can lead to much trouble in life – an attitude of meaninglessness and a loss of motivation to engage in living. The very act of affirming *non-duality* (unmanifest *Oneness*) and the non-existence of *duality* (*Oneness* plus diversity) can lead to a sense of hopelessness if one is not experiencing at least a smidgen of the thing itself, the witness.

It is like asking a bird who is yet to grow wings to jump off the top of a building. The bird with fully developed and functioning wings will keep saying to the one with undeveloped wings, "Come on, you can do it. Just jump. Don't worry about the wings."

Does this make any sense? The wings have to come first. Then we can fly.

It is time to face up to the fact that one size of self-inquiry does not fit all. Cookbook self-inquiry in the form of mental algorithms and formula thinking does not work for everyone.

Rather, self-inquiry is a continuum that is tied to the level of inner silence we are experiencing as a known presence within us. It is the witness. That is the real thing. That is the blank screen behind the movie of life.

When we engage in self-inquiry from that position, then we will have a relationship between consciousness (our witness) and the idea. Then there can be an intimate cognition in silence of the reality conveyed by the idea. This is knowledge.

On the other hand, if we are identified largely with our thoughts, and perceive these to be our self, then the idea of our thoughts will be interacting with the idea of our self – two ideas interacting with each other. Castles in the air. In this case there is no intimate relationship between consciousness and the idea. It is all happening in the mind.

It is important to understand these two situations, and how a natural shift will occur as we, as the witness, move into true relationship with our thoughts, feelings, and perceptions of the surroundings, leading to direct cognition of who and what we are. If we develop clarity about what the maneuvering of our mind is and what our true presence is, then we will find ourselves going beyond all objects, including our thoughts. We will be going beyond the mental processes of self-inquiry as well, which is the only true self-inquiry – *That* which dissolves thinking immediately with the first question, and *That* which inhabits all answers with stillness. Of course, this is made possible by cultivating the witness in daily deep meditation.

In order to better gage where we are, it can be helpful to designate parameters to describe where we may be in our efforts to engage in self-inquiry. Such designations would not be necessary if all who entered into self-inquiry were coming from the same place – the point of view of the inner witness. However, this is not the case, so making some distinctions can be helpful.

The truth is that much of the self-inquiry that goes on these days is *non-relational* (meaning, not progressive) and often counter-productive to spiritual progress, because it adds layers of mental baggage without much cultivation of our native awareness. Ironically, effective practices which do cultivate the witness may be shunned in favor of such a rigid approach, which does not cultivate a relationship between the objects of perception and the witness. So much of self-inquiry today is like this, and many find themselves beating their head against a wall. It isn't necessary!

On the other hand, for the few who have had abiding inner silence since an early age, there will nearly always be a relationship between ideas and infinite awareness. Self-inquiry in this case is *relational*. These are the spontaneously awakened souls who dazzle us with their insight, and who are often idolized and imitated. There is an air of exclusivity about them, which can unintentionally lead to a *have or have not* mentality.

Enlightenment is not an exclusive condition reserved for the few, and the rest of us are not doomed to imitate the instruction to "Just be." No. With the addition of deep meditation and other practices that promote the cultivation of the witness, and much more, self-inquiry will be *relational* and the direct cognition of life as a dance of endless joy in emptiness will be there for everyone.

By *relational self-inquiry*, we mean a progressive and intimate relationship between ideas and our inner consciousness. When our thoughts are naturally witnessed as objects, something happens. A joining occurs, and the idea dissolves along with its meaning in stillness. Then we will know the truth of it.

For example, if we ask the question, *"Who am I?"* and let go into our stillness, the answer will be there, not as an idea, but as part of us in presence. We will know who we are beyond the surroundings, our body, thoughts and feelings. If we have been cultivating inner silence in daily deep meditation, the answer will be there to an increasing degree over time, until eventually all that we have known to be *other* will be dancing on our field of awareness like waves on the unmoving depths of the ocean.

On the other hand, if we go about mentally chanting, *"Who am I? Who am I? Who am I?!"* pounding the idea away without any significant stillness or presence of the witness, without any letting go, then this will be *non-relational self-inquiry*. It can lead to a lot of frustration, and real headaches. Much better to get behind all that by developing our inner quality of stillness, which we can then let go into easily when engaged in self-inquiry.

In our daily activities and relationships, we may be inclined to inquire about the nature of the experiences and interactions we encounter. If someone becomes angry with us, and we find ourselves responding in kind, we may inquire, *"Is my rising anger based in truth?"* and then let it go into stillness. If we are abiding in the witness, the answer will be there. We will know that our negative reactions are rooted in our identification with the body-mind, which we have falsely regarded as our self. As we become identified with the anger of another, we may be inclined to mirror that. But is that the truth? Can't we just as easily mirror the anger of another with a loving reply? What have we got to lose but the anger itself? The abiding witness gives us the ability to make that choice, where before the witness we could only react to negative energy in kind. The witness puts us in the position of having a choice, and when we have that choice, we have the option to take the high road.

Life operates on knee-jerks, on habits and *dramatic stories* that have been deeply ingrained in us for a long time. We draw our conclusions about every situation in life based on these habits. It is like we are the hero in our drama and everyone else is the potential enemy. It doesn't have to be this way. As we begin to see the world and ourselves from the perspective of our own inner silence, we will also see that we can change our reactions to things. We will be compelled to do so, because the truth rising within us does not mesh with the untrue habits we have been unintentionally expressing in so many ways. So we begin to make different choices about how we act, based on what we are actually seeing.

Oddly, if we project this divine process of choosing beyond where we are in stillness in the present, there will be strain. As soon as we do that, we will find ourselves slipping into non-relational self-inquiry, building more mental structures, often in ways we may not even recognize. Relationship is letting go. Non-relationship is hanging on, including hanging on to letting go!

It is the difference between theory and practice. Theory is thinking about doing, and practice is the doing itself. So much of self-inquiry out there is only about theory, about philosophy. Real self-inquiry is about practice, about the thing itself, which is engaging as the witness.

Why bother with all this relational and non-relational mumbo-jumbo? It is suggested not to bother with it much. We don't want to be adding too much mental baggage. Just recognize that self-inquiry is not about doing, projecting or protecting. It is about going beyond the machinations of the mind with simple questions and automatic answers that rise in stillness – easily favoring the stillness within. Our ability to do this is directly related to the degree of inner silence we have present. So be sure to take care of the business of cultivating inner silence before engaging in self-inquiry. Then you will be flying on the wings of the witness.

Five Stages of Mind

There are many schools of self-inquiry, embodying a variety of systems of practice. Each may emphasize a particular angle, with its own philosophy, terminology and mental algorithms.

The methods can vary widely, from prescribing complete conscious engagement (mindfulness) in the minutest details of life, to letting go of life altogether. Whatever the teaching may be, it will always reflect the experience of the particular teacher who is transmitting the knowledge. There will be a bias, and the teaching may or may not resonate with all students who come to study that approach. When a student does not *get it*, it is usually regarded to be the shortcoming of the student, not the teaching itself, which is often held as immutable.

Well, perhaps the end result is immutable, the realization of the eternal within the student. But if the teaching does not help open the door, it can only be the teaching that is failing, not the student. This is a common problem with teachings that are fixed, held high up on a pedestal, and not adaptable for students coming in at many different levels of readiness.

Of what use are such teachings to the masses in modern times? They are from a past era when only the few were regarded to be worthy of spiritual knowledge. The fact is, only those who were near enlightenment already were capable of gaining much from such teachings. And those few likely would have finished the task of human spiritual transformation, regardless.

Times are changing. Now it is time for spiritual teachings to serve the people, instead of the other way around. And in order to do so, the teachings must be open, flexible, and, most importantly, effective. To be effective, such teachings must be capable of addressing every student at every level of readiness. If the student has the desire to grow and is willing to make a commitment of time and some discipline, then the teaching must be able to deliver viable means, or it will be in need of some improvement. This is okay. If teachings are flexible, they will learn to serve the people where they are, and evolve as the people evolve.

Self-inquiry is a particularly tricky one for application for different levels of students. In our case, we will begin with daily deep meditation, which will cultivate inner silence in everyone. Additional methods of yoga will be added as appropriate. A foundational knowledge of self-inquiry will also be necessary.

First, it is good to know that in our essential nature we are unbounded pure bliss consciousness, and that all we are doing in practices is unfolding what we already are in our daily life. It is also good to know that this will lead to many practical benefits. So, it is a worthwhile endeavor to be on the path.

Next, it is also good to know that there is a natural progression in our spiritual unfoldment which occurs over time, usually over a long time, except in the rare cases of people who are born near enlightenment. In spite of what we may have heard, enlightenment is not an overnight event for most people. There is no getting around this, because each of us must go through a process of inner purification and opening, and it takes time, even with the best of teachings. Along the way, there are grades and stages, and the journey never ends, even for those who are very advanced. Perhaps especially for them, because they become much more aware of the wider need for rising inner silence in the community, world and beyond, and find themselves on the front line of that great endeavor. We all help as we can, and the enlightened can help so much more. The more we can do, the more we will be called to do.

For the individual, there is a progression of integrated practices that is mapped out in a step-by-step way in the over all *Advanced Yoga Practices* (AYP) writings, for cultivating the necessary purification and opening. For self-inquiry, there is a progression also. Not that it is required for everyone to go through a progression of self-inquiry methods. One may not even use structured self-inquiry methods at all, and still be going through the process of self-inquiry based on the natural emergence of inner silence and the increasingly clear perceptions of *Self* in relation to the objects of experience. Regardless of structured self-inquiry methods, or the lack of them, some recognizable stages will evolve, and it can save time and some confusion to be aware of these, particularly for those ,who have a tendency to try and run to the end before covering the beginning or the middle. The beginning and the middle can be just as fulfilling as the end if we are reasonably well in touch with where we are on our path. It does not have to be so mysterious. With some basic knowledge, we will do much better, and not be so much exposed to the hazards of taking blind leaps.

Assuming one is engaged in daily deep meditation, here are five stages of mind that self-inquiry may play itself upon as we move along in our development:

1. Pre-Witnessing – Information and intellectual assessments about truth provide inspiration, and a tendency to build mental castles in the air, ideas reacting with ideas, which is non-relational self-inquiry. So we do what is necessary to cultivate the witness.

2. Witnessing – Perceiving the world, our thoughts and feelings as objects separate from *Self*. It is the beginning of relational self-inquiry, chosen or not.

3. Discrimination – The reversal of identification by logical choices based on direct perception rooted in stillness. This is more advanced relational self-inquiry which is able to discern the real from the unreal.

4. Dispassion – Rise of the condition of no judgment and no attachment. The process of self-inquiry becoming automatic to the point of all objects and self-inquiry itself being constantly dissolved in the witness.

5. Merging of Subject and Object – "I am *That*. You are *That*. All this is *That*." Ongoing outpouring divine love, service to others, and unity.

While progress on the road to enlightenment may be erratic, difficult or non-existent when engaged in self-inquiry as a stand-alone approach, it is quite a different story when self-inquiry is used in concert with a path based on an integration of tried and true yoga methods.

The cultivation of inner silence (the witness) in deep meditation assures that our perception will be expanding from within over time, and this provides for an increasingly fertile field for the process of self-inquiry to occur.

The steady emergence of inner silence with practices is the dynamic behind the progression of self-inquiry from non-relational to relational, until the experiencer and the experience have merged to become the *One*.

Pre-Witnessing

How meaningful is self-inquiry of the absolute kind when we are still in the pre-witnessing stage of mind? This is when all things are still considered primarily on the level of thinking and logic. In this state, what does it mean to us when we hear, "All this you see here in the world is illusion, and you are the reality behind it."

We might have some inspiration, a desire may be kindled to know more, to be more. Hopefully. But the more we think about it, the more layers we will create around that essential desire to know the truth. How many times will we have to repeat the question *"Who am I?"* before we will have a glimmer of who and what we really are? And how many books will we have to read? This is why we call pre-witnessing the stage of *inspiration and building castles in the air*. Not much more than this can happen until we move to the next stage. With suitable inspiration, we will be compelled to take action beyond pounding the idea against the infinite with our tiny brain!

Once we are inspired to uncover the truth, it is important to take action, intelligent action. Self-inquiry purists will say, "Take no action. Do nothing. Just be!" Well, we can attempt to do that for a very long time in pre-witnessing mode. No doubt we can develop some witness quality by working on just being for a long time. But there is a much faster way.

If we commit to take action using all the tools that are available to us, we can travel very quickly along the road of realizing what we already are – our inner most *Self.* With deep meditation and a full battery of supporting practices we will move surely into the witnessing stage.

Witnessing

The witnessing stage is a whole new ball game. It should be pointed out that there is witnessing and there is witnessing. There is a continuum of development as witnessing emerges. It begins as a passive inner condition perceived as a separation from the events going on around us, often first noticed during the occurrence of dynamic events. Everyone has had the experience of *time standing still* when a dynamic event occurred, like a car crash, explosion or other sudden change in our physical environment. When the witness begins to emerge, ordinary events are gradually experienced more in this way also. As witnessing continues to advance, our body, thoughts and feelings become objects of perception that are separate from our sense of self, our witness. This is an important development.

Before the witness has developed to the point where our thoughts and feelings become objects of perception, self-inquiry will be mostly non-relational, meaning not fully connected with who we are – pure consciousness. The dawn of the witness sets the stage for real self-inquiry, and an ongoing change in our life experience, for this is when the process can move beyond ideas to the direct experience. And the direct experience is *beyond* all experience. In the initial witness condition, we are experiencing, but we are not the experience. We are beyond it, seeing from the point of view of separate pure awareness.

There are a few more steps beyond the emergence of the witness that we must go through. It is not enough to be strongly established in the inner silence, seeing the changing world as separate from ourselves. We must do something with it to move it forward. Evolution compels us to do so. With a little nudging, it happens naturally enough. This is where self-inquiry can have its greatest impact on our over all path to enlightenment, because we are able to make conscious choices based in our stillness. We see our thoughts, feelings and perceptions of the world for what they are, without being entirely identified with them. We are then able to engage in a way that is liberating rather than binding, both for ourselves and for others.

Discrimination

When we think of discrimination, the normal interpretation is that we are choosing between this or that thing – choosing between this or that idea. Non-relational self-inquiry is like that, choosing between things, ideas, and ways we imagine we would like for life to be. This kind of discrimination goes nowhere fast, and may go nowhere for a long time. Even choosing not to think is a gigantic task when undertaken non-relationally, without the witness present to support our endeavor.

With the rising presence of the witness, the entire dynamic of self-inquiry changes. Then we are choosing between that which is object (things, ideas, emotions) and that which is subject (witness, *Self*). And that kind of choosing is not a doing at all. It is a letting go.

We all know what we want. We want to know the truth. We want to be happy. We want to be free. Since childhood we have been told that the truth will set us free from the burdens of this life. So we want *That*.

As the witness becomes more and more abiding and we come to know ourselves as *That*, unshaken and separate from all of our experiences, including our own thoughts, then we are finally in the position to make choices that will unwind the habitual identification with experiences and the dream we have been in up until now.

It is a new perspective from which we can clearly see what is real and what is not. At the same time, it is both as profound and as simple as directly perceiving what is eternal and what is not. And we can discriminate accordingly, making logical choices that are grounded in stillness, unwinding the lingering habit of the mind to identify itself with the objects of experience, both outside and inside us.

In the language of yoga, it is called *neti neti*, which means *not this and not this*. When the witness is sufficiently present for relational self-inquiry to occur in the form of discrimination, then neti neti becomes a reality. We directly perceive what is true and what is not, and we can easily choose. Before then, neti neti will be an exercise of the intellect, and can be as ineffective and exhausting as any other non-relational self-inquiry. We will know the witness is dawning in earnest when discrimination becomes easier. It is a telltale sign.

A certain excitement comes with the realization that we have arrived at the point of being able to choose with certainty that which is real over that which is not.

There can even be an enthusiasm to the exclusion of all else, and we have to guard against throwing out the practices that have brought us to this point. There can be a strong tendency to plant our flag on the notion that we are *That*, and fixating on the idea that all we have to do from then on is hang onto *That*.

If this happens, it can be slipping into non-relational self-inquiry again. It can happen to advanced practitioners. Much better we should continue with the practices that brought us to this point and strengthen the presence of the witness beyond all tendencies we might have to imagine that we have attained anything. Even the most advanced practitioners must guard against falling into non-relational self-inquiry.

Certainly we can take giant leaps toward realization when our ability has arisen to clearly discriminate between objects (external and internal) and the subject (the witness – our *Self*). It is prime time for self-inquiry. But it will not be the only thing going on, assuming we have been wise and continue with our daily routine of yoga practices. All methods combined will assure our rapid forward progress.

Self-inquiry is useful, but it cannot be trusted to operate alone. Certainly not at the discrimination stage, or at any prior stage.

There will come a time when discrimination begins to give way to something else. It is the letting go of the need to make choices anymore. The subject (witness) becomes so well established that choices no longer need to be made. We just are, and we can allow everything in our field of awareness to just be, even as we are interacting normally in every day living. We call this the dispassion stage. It is the stage of being completely unruffled by anything that happens inside or outside us.

Dispassion

The condition of dispassion is one of the primary goals of self-inquiry. Those who are very enthusiastic and dedicated to self-inquiry are very passionate about developing dispassion. This is non-relational self-inquiry, of course.

Dispassion is not a doing at all, and is beyond self-inquiry itself. It isn't even a letting go, for it is beyond choice. Dispassion is a state of being. It is the subject (the witness, our sense of *Self*) developed through an integration of practices to the point where all the objects of experience are taken in stride, without identification. This applies to events, relationships, and all that is going on in the body, heart and mind.

Is dispassion a state of indifference, a state of uncaring? Does it mean we do not act or react in the world? It does not mean that. It is just the opposite. Much of spiritual development is paradoxical, with less becoming much more.

The gradual emergence of dispassion means we are becoming more free to act for the good of all. Inner silence will *move* to do this through us more and more, the further we travel along the path. It is the paradox of enlightenment. The more we have gone beyond, the more engaged we will become for the benefit of others. This is the nature of divine consciousness.

We really have to give credit where credit is due. Deep meditation (if we are doing it) is the primary cultivator of dispassion, because dispassion is an advanced stage of the witness. A stand-alone path of self-inquiry can lead to dispassion also, but it is rare. To succeed, self-inquiry must ascend to the level of meditation, the transcendence of all objects of attention. If self-inquiry is done like this over time, then witness will dawn and, in more time, there wi dispassion. It is a difficult path, because it lacks a structured and efficient routine of practice (like twice-daily deep meditation). The concept of *practice* itself may be lacking. Self-inquiry of the stand-alone variety will be about constantly remembering to disregard/release all objects of perception, including all thoughts, feelings and perceptions of external objects. When self-inquiry becomes a deeply ingrained habit, then that will be a kind of ongoing meditation. How an approach like this will fit into daily life is another question, since it requires ongoing self-inquiry to be incorporated into every nook and cranny of our daily life. This may not be practical for someone with a family and career. There can be direct conflicts, particularly before the witness has dawned.

On the other hand, if deep meditation is undertaken in a structured twice-daily routine, and life is lived normally, the witness will be coming up naturally as a support to family and career, and also as a support to undertake self-inquiry in a way that does not disrupt the normal flow of life. Deep meditation provides the witness and self-inquiry provides the perspective in a way that is not replacing every day life and activities, but enhancing them.

Dispassion is at home in the marketplace, as well as in the remote retreat. It is all the same. The combination of daily deep meditation and gradually emerging self-inquiry provides much more flexibility for living, and is a much faster path as well.

ng Divine Love and Unity

ws what the true nature of existence is
f time and space. Yet, oddly enough,
e it directly. The reason we say "We
because the reality we are all able to

experience through deep meditation and self-inquiry is outside the field of knowing. It is *That*, and thousands of volumes have been written attempting to describe *That*.

In the end, the best we can do is say, "I am *That*." Then we can carry on with the many descriptions of *That* – pure bliss consciousness, void, Tao, God, Allah… It doesn't really matter what we call it. *That* is as good a word as any, and we are *That*. All that exists is *That*.

If it sounds a little impersonal, it is not intended to be. For *That* is the source of all love, compassion, goodness, creativity and happiness in the world. *That* illuminates us with these divine qualities, and is the source of all good deeds.

There is a misunderstanding that has been perpetuated by some teachers – the premise that becoming *That* is the only thing of importance and nothing here on earth matters at all. In fact, according to this premise, nothing here on earth exists. In a philosophical sense this may be true. We also learned it in high school quantum physics, yes? Yet, when taken on the level of intellect, it is one of the biggest traps for getting stuck in non-relational self-inquiry.

There is the idea that it matters not one bit what becomes of this earth or the multitude of life that is on it. There is a distinction between one who is truly enlightened and one who has created a division between themselves and the rest of the world through non-relational self-inquiry, enforced by a rigid intellectual view. With clear relational self-inquiry based in stillness, we can reject this out of hand. *Neti neti!*

The enlightened one will be he or she who remains engaged for the benefit of all, as *That*. Advancement on the path to enlightenment brings with it the perception that we can only be free when all are free, for we are *One* with all that exists.

The image of the lone sage on the mountaintop, indifferent to the travails of the world, is fiction. If a sage is not engaged for the benefit of others, their condition will be in question. True enlightenment is the spontaneous outpouring of divine love, which is working constantly to uplift everyone. The sage becomes a willing and wide open channel for *That*, which does nothing while doing everything.

So, while yoga and self-inquiry are often viewed as a going beyond, never to return, it is not so. We can never leave what is here and now, for it is what we are in our own *Self*. The journey of yoga, and of self-inquiry, is a journey beyond all that is, ending in a return and full engagement for the betterment of humankind – a journey from *here to here*. This is the highest knowledge, and its highest manifestation in this world.

"I am That. You are That. All this is That."

It is an unending outpouring of divine love, whose fundamental nature and fruition is life everywhere residing in the *Oneness* of unity. It has always been *That* and will always be *That*. The witness and self-inquiry lead to direct realization of *That*.

Honoring Our Nature and Where We Are

Everyone has different inclinations and tendencies about how to live their life. This is also true in spiritual matters. Each of us has our path already built into our own nature. All we must do is tread it. Easier said than done.

Advice will be coming from all directions, especially as our spiritual desire (bhakti) is rising. When the student is ready, the teacher will appear. More likely many teachers!

It is up to us to honor our nature and where we happen to be on our path, and proceed accordingly. In the AYP writings, we call this *self-pacing*, which is a very important component when undertaking any spiritual practice.

Self-pacing is particularly important when considering self-inquiry, because it is easy to fall into a non-relational self-inquiry practice that will not be serving our best interest. This will be any self-inquiry practice that is not in harmony with our *inner call*, which is a direct expression of inner silence (the witness) coming out through our unique nature. Even with a strong inner desire to engage in self-inquiry, some common sense should be incorporated to regulate our efforts in a way to assure smooth and safe progress on our path.

Not everyone will be called to self-inquiry in the beginning. If our heart calls us to dance the night away for God, or to be engaged in service to others, what good will it be to deny the relevance or existence of these heartfelt urges within us? We can dance, and we can serve! Self-inquiry will enter into our spiritual life in a way that is appropriate for us, if we allow it to happen without forcing. We will see the transcendent unmoving divine playing in every joyous act.

On the other hand, if we are contemplative and quiet in our nature, we may be inclined to engage in self-inquiry more than those who may lean toward a more devotional expression.

In either case, we will be wise to be engaging in daily deep meditation, so the witness will be dawning from within, no matter what our tendencies might be in life. That way, self-inquiry will find a fertile field upon which to manifest that which is appropriate for us as we go about our daily activities. Then we will be able to interpret the truth of the world as we are living it according to our own nature.

In general, it is not a good idea to try and live our life according to the dictates of someone else, particularly if our inner voice is telling us that something is not right in the circumstance we may find ourselves in.

It is also important to honor our inherent nature and inner dynamics as they relate to the process of purification and opening that will be occurring as we engage in practices. This is an essential aspect of regulating sitting practices such as deep meditation, spinal breathing pranayama, samyama, mudras, bandhas, and so on. Self-pacing is readily addressed by temporarily scaling back on the time of a practice if symptoms of purification related to that practice become excessive and uncomfortable. With daily practices, the nervous system will go through a process of purification, and our job is to manage practices in a way that will sustain steady progress with comfort and safety.

Self-pacing for self-inquiry is a bit more complicated, because most of us will not be doing it according to a predetermined schedule. Chances are, self-inquiry will be happening either naturally in relation to the rise of our inner witness, or in a deliberate way that may have little relationship to the degree of inner silence we have. There is a chance for overdoing and excessive purification and discomfort in using self-inquiry in either case.

Relational self-inquiry (with the witness) will tend to be less disruptive, even if overdone a bit. Even so, we will be wise to scale back on self-inquiry and do other things (like take long walks or other *grounding* activities) if we begin to feel off center or overdone. In the latter case of overdoing in non-relational self-inquiry (with limited witness), there can be headaches, dizziness, disorientation, depression, lethargy in every day activity, and a loss of motivation to pursue our goals in life. In the case of overdoing non-relational self-inquiry, the symptoms can be very destabilizing.

So, we will be wise to keep an eye on how we feel in going about our daily activities. If our sitting practices are in balance, and our self-inquiry is relational and not excessive, then we will find increasing peace and joy in life, and we will be less inclined to find ourselves in the grip of suffering, even in adverse circumstances. If our practices, including self-inquiry, are not in balance, we will notice symptoms related to the extra strain we are creating, and it is suggested to scale back accordingly until we find smoothness in daily activity returning.

Everyone will be a little different in this. If we honor our nature and where we are on our path, then our progress on the way to realization will be steady, with fewer disruptions along the way.

Chapter 3 – Self-Inquiry in Daily Life

It is becoming clear by now that self-inquiry is a more tricky business than doing our sitting practices twice each day like clockwork. We know that if we are engaging in deep meditation daily, then the stillness of the inner witness will be coming up in every aspect of our life, and that this will open many doors for us. We will become more peaceful, more creative and happier in whatever we happen to be doing. This has been the experience of many.

Self-inquiry is not like this, or at least there is not reliable evidence to this effect. What we do know about self-inquiry is that there is a lot of interest in it. Its appealing logic is a magnet for the mind. We also know that self-inquiry is something best done in-between our sitting practice sessions, which can be a small or large part of our day. With the rise of the witness, self-inquiry can be a natural thing as we go about our daily activities, just easily noticing what is true and what is not as our perception expands.

But many of us will be looking for more than that sort of natural emergence of self-inquiry, which is an automatic discrimination. The mind loves to analyze, and it is more inclined to hang on than let go. So, looking at the role of self-inquiry in daily living is as much about what it is not as it is about what it is.

Much of what people are doing in self-inquiry in daily living these days is the result of what teachers have written and said. So let's look first at the role of the teacher in this. Then we can broaden it out to look at what actually constitutes self-inquiry in daily living, and what does not.

Teachers – Pros and Cons

These days, there seems to be an abundance of *spontaneously realized* teachers crisscrossing the landscape. They are more than willing to share with us what it is like to see the world through their eyes, and many are naturally inclined to offer stand-alone self-inquiry approaches, because this is how they see the world – a superimposition of the unreal upon the real. So, from their point of view, all that is necessary is for everyone to make the distinction between real and unreal – the problem of ignorance solved in an instant.

Such teachers are sincere in their sharing, wanting to help us find a way beyond our identification with this world, beyond our dream, and beyond seeking itself. However, there is a difficulty in following what these teachers offer. We can see where they are and where we are, but the means for traveling from here to there is not always clear.

Spontaneously realized teachers may say things like:

"Let go. Be here now. None of this is real. Keep asking '*Who am I?*' and '*Who is experiencing this?*' Know the world to be emptiness with no substance. There is nothing here and there is nothing to do. Therefore, spiritual practices are not necessary."

This is the classic *advaita* (non-dual) approach to self-inquiry and spiritual development. In fact, it professes no spiritual development at all. Only the unmanifest reality beyond the ups and downs of this life is regarded as real, and we are *That* already, to the exclusion of all else, even the many means available to aid in that very realization.

While philosophically sound, on the practical level it is a narrow view, which contains more than a little irony – the exclusion of the world from an all-inclusive non-dual view! A growing throng of modern spiritual teachers stand as proof of the fact. So why are so few of us benefiting from this approach?

Assuming a realized teacher of this type has charisma and credibility, the result of this kind of teaching will often lead to imitation of the teacher, rather than cultivating the realization itself. The buzz will be mainly about the teacher and not about the student. This may happen in spite of the wishes of the teacher. That's just how it is. To the extent real spiritual experience does occur in the student, it may be short-lived (and sometimes chaotic) if practical means are not offered to expand and stabilize it in daily living.

While there can be much inspiration in visiting and listening to spontaneously realized teachers, if they do not offer a structured and effective daily practice that can easily blend with the modern lifestyle, then the long term value of what they are offering will be open to question.

The truth is that the majority of advaita/non-duality-style teachers, past and present, have taught *non-relational* self-inquiry. Not because they wanted to, but because their students have not had enough presence of the witness to make self-inquiry effective beyond the initial shivers of instinctive recognition. Any *relational* self-inquiry that has been occurring has been a result of how much inner silence the student has brought to the table in the first place, rather than the particular brand of self-inquiry being offered by the teacher.

When it comes to self-inquiry, the magic formula is not found in the method itself. It is found in the degree of abiding witness in the student. And that is the product of the conduct of effective spiritual practices (especially meditation), either recently or in times long past and forgotten.

Many spiritual teachers miss this point, because they teach from the perspective of their own level of experience. This can lead to a situation like a master mathematician attempting to teach calculus to grammar school students. What good will the calculus be if the students have not yet learned how to add and subtract? If the gap between the teacher and student is not closed somehow, progress will be limited. This is the situation when realized teachers attempt to teach self-inquiry to students who have not been given the opportunity to cultivate the witness.

Self-inquiry is not rocket science. When the witness is present, self-inquiry occurs naturally as an *effect*, based on direct perception of the transcendental *Self* (the witness) in relation to our perception of thoughts, feelings and the objects of the world. To cultivate this kind of subject-object relationship with self-inquiry alone is very difficult. If it were not difficult, we would have many more enlightened people running around, and many fewer people stuck at the feet of the realized, hoping for an awakening by osmosis. It doesn't work like that – not for long.

This situation is sometimes blamed on the student not being ready for the "highest teaching," which advaita/non-duality is held to be. While the philosophy and the realization itself can be said to be the highest, the teaching certainly is not. If the means for developing the essential prerequisite for self-inquiry are not being provided by the teacher, it is not the student's failing, but the teacher's. That essential prerequisite is the *witness*.

The highest teaching is not necessarily the one with the highest ideal or objective. All spiritual teachings aspire to more or less the same ideal – the direct realization of ultimate truth, or God. But there is a huge difference in approaches, and this is where the distinction should be made on what is highest. Not on the end goal, which will always be the same.

From this point of view, the highest teaching is the one that enables the most people to directly realize the truth of existence quickly and easily.

The highest teaching is one that is the most effective and accessible for everyone. This will not necessarily be the most structured teaching, but one that is flexible and facilitates individual expression while being solidly grounded in the underlying principles of self-inquiry, meaning, the establishment of the witness and its relationship with the machinery of perception.

It is vitally important for every spiritual teacher to meet their students where they are with practical means that are appropriate for them at their present level of development.

As we come into a time when there is much more integration of methodologies occurring across traditional lines, more teachers are incorporating meditation in combination with the methods of self-inquiry. It is a logical step, and one that is much needed to cover the full range of students, and break the log-jam of non-relational self-inquiry. It is not a great distance from non-relational to relational self-inquiry. It is only a witness away.

So, while realized teachers can provide a lot of inspiration, we need much more from them. Most important are practical means that students can take home with them for enhancing their experience in daily life. Then the truth will be accessible to everyone, and can be directly perceived and further revealed through the natural application of self-inquiry methods in daily living.

It is important to recognize that no matter how much spiritual energy teachers may give us in the form of inspiration, inner stimulation, or intellectual knowledge, the greatest value will come from our daily practices over the long term. If they give us a routine that will carry us steadily forward day by day into a direct realization of our true nature, without turning our life upside down in the process, then they will have done their job.

It is the duty of all students to demand nothing less from spiritual teachers. If a teacher cannot or will not deliver effective means, then it will be wise to look beyond for additional sources of knowledge.

All teachings have benefit, but no teaching covers all aspects of the process of human spiritual transformation. So it is good to keep an open mind, and be willing to make the choices that are necessary to move ahead. No teacher can make these choices for us. We have to take responsibility for our own spiritual progress.

The greatest teacher is within us.

Practical Applications of Self-Inquiry

We know now that self-inquiry is practical when it is relational, and not very practical when it is non-relational. What does this mean?

If we are inquiring about who we are (*Who am I?*), or making affirmations about who we are (I am *That*), and these are only ideas making more ideas, rather than releasing into the actual presence of inner silence (the witness), then the inquiry or affirmation will be non-relational, and therefore not very practical. From this, it stands to reason that the level and kind of self-inquiry we are doing will, by necessity, be matched up with the degree of witness we have present in our awareness. The more prevalent the witness, the more far-reaching our self-inquiry will be, while remaining relational.

So, logically, the first step on a path of self-inquiry will be the ongoing cultivation of the witness. In the approach we use in AYP, that will be via deep meditation. In any effective system where self-inquiry is employed, some kind of meditation will be present, whether it be in the form of a regular sitting practice, or an aspect of the self-inquiry itself.

Once we have been cultivating the witness, the next step will be to notice its presence. It may be noticed as a calmness – events occurring without leaving impressions as they did before, more happiness, a bubbling up of creative energy, increased desire to know the truth via more study and inquiry. Or we may notice a silent wakefulness in-between our waking thoughts, during dreaming while we are asleep, or while we are in dreamless deep sleep. Any or all of these.

Once we have noticed the witness, we may still find the absolute philosophical tenet of non-duality to be quite foreign – the idea that there is only *That*, and all this I experience in the world and in my mind is illusion, unreal. Hammering on this idea will not help us much to see that it is so, though anyone is welcome to do that. It will likely remain non-relational for some time before the truth begins to peek through.

Much better to continue with daily sitting practices, and then take on self-inquiry right where we are in more mundane ways. If we learn to crawl first, and then stand up while holding on to something, we will be much less likely to fall flat on our face when we try to walk. If we take it step-by-step, we will be running before we know it. At some point we may find ourselves having the time to *notice who is noticing*. It doesn't take any time at all really – only the witness. It begins in the many gaps of stillness that occur in-between everything that happens in our daily experience, between our thoughts, feelings and perceptions of the world. Eventually, the gaps expand and merge to encompass our experience twenty-four hours per day. Then we notice our stillness has become the blank movie screen upon which the entire drama of life is being projected.

Let's consider the five stages of mind discussed in the previous chapter. When we get to the point where we begin to witness our surroundings, thoughts, and feelings as being somehow outside ourselves (see last chapter, stage 2 – witnessing), then this is not necessarily the time to drop our active engagement in the world in favor of asserting, "I am *That*!"

It isn't necessarily the time either for pressing hard in our every waking moment with the inquiry, "*Who am I?*" While noticing and becoming identified with the witness puts us in the position to discriminate between the objects of our perception and the witness (stage 3), it does not mean we are ready to jump straight into dispassion (stage 4) and full realization of "I am *That*" (stage 5). It would be nice, but it seldom works that way. For those who try and leap that far immediately when they find a taste of real discrimination, it can be a rocky road with a lot of confusion and non-relational backsliding. Or is it forward sliding?

Either way, instead of taking the leap, we will be wise to inquire about our every day experiences in the here and now first, and begin to find relational self-inquiry in those. By bringing in the witness through daily deep meditation and gradually taking a different tact in our relationship with our own thoughts, we can improve our effectiveness and happiness in daily living. This kind of self-inquiry has tangible benefits, and is worth doing. Then we will be on our way to a more ultimate kind of self-inquiry. There is a natural progression in it.

We all know how difficult it can be to change our life by thinking alone, and some of us struggle with it constantly. It seems no matter how hard we try, our relationships seem to keep going along the same tracks, and the realization we are working to achieve may elude us for a long time. The reason is because we are wrapped up in the ways we relate and in the ways we pursue our objectives in life. In short, we are *identified* with the life we have been living, including our style of thinking and relating. Deep inside, we believe that this is who we are.

The witness is beyond these deep-seated beliefs, so when we begin to inquire from that perspective, the identification begins to unwind. Then we begin to see beyond our dream, and can interact in ways that may have seemed impossible to us before.

Freedom! It is very practical.

We don't have to worry about realizing the ultimate truth, because once we begin to get our every day house in order with relational self-inquiry, the big picture will not be far from us. It is important to avoid over-extending ourselves. We should learn to stand up and walk before we try and run.

There is great truth in the advice that if we want to measure the merit of a sage, we should look first at their ordinary relationships, rather than at their mystical attainments.

There are a variety of self-inquiry systems and they fall into two categories:

- Inquiry about our every day interactions and activities, with the aim to live in greater harmony and happiness.

- Inquiry about the ultimate nature of existence, and who we are in relation to *That*.

To be honest, the various kinds of self-inquiry systems in these two categories will work equally well if the witness is present. If there is a grain of truth in them, the witness will know, and self-inquiry will be good. Even if there is only little truth in a particular angle of inquiry, the witness will find the truth in that also. All inquiry for truth, whether on the level of every day living or the cosmic level, depends on that kind of resonance with truth (the witness). The presence of that resonance in self-inquiry is what makes it relational and practical.

Not everyone is inclined to engage in structured self-inquiry, using specific mental algorithms, or formulas. That is okay. Structured self-inquiry is not mandatory if we are cultivating the witness. Our ongoing desire for truth and the presence of the witness will be enough to bring us along into full realization in good time. In that situation, we will know the truth, whether we are deliberately inquiring or not.

Ironically, those who are the most enthusiastic about doing self-inquiry will often be those who will gain the least from it. These are people with very curious and analytical minds, constantly testing mental algorithms, but perhaps with less inclination to bring the mind to stillness in daily deep meditation. So there will be a lot of *non-relational* inquiry and analysis going on there, but very little *relational* self-inquiry.

There are numerous systems of self-inquiry that are offered in the spiritual marketplace these days. All will be effective if they are done relationally, with presence of the witness. And not one of them will be effective if it is done non-relationally, with thoughts manipulating and interacting with thoughts. For this reason, we are not laying out specific schemes of structured self-inquiry in detail here. The effectiveness of self-inquiry does not rely very much on the particular mental algorithm we happen to be using.

Therefore, it is not necessary to examine the many structured systems of self-inquiry in this small book. It will be easy enough to look them up and gravitate toward approaches that suit our nature. Or perhaps we will evolve our own way of inquiring deep into the nature of things in relation to the rise of our own witness consciousness. In self-inquiry especially, the natural approach is usually the best approach, because it carries no pretense. We call it as we see it. We will know the approach to self-inquiry we are using is *relational* by its ease and effectiveness.

Until we have found our own way by direct experience in stillness, this book can be a help in understanding the underlying principles of self-inquiry, and put us in a better position to evaluate any system of self-inquiry, or any philosophy and its mental strategies for unfolding full human potential. In taking a wise approach by cultivating the witness first, we will be able to easily distinguish useful methods from those that are not so useful for us at every step along the way. We will find the truth everywhere when we have the inner witness to see it.

In discussing self-inquiry here, we will make a fundamental distinction between how we regard our every day experiences, and how we might regard the ultimate truth of existence and our role in it. These are different categories of self-inquiry directly related to the stages of mind discussed in the last chapter. Both are essentially about the same thing, and are leading to the same realization.

Self-Inquiry for Every Day Experiences

Once the witness is dawning, we will be inclined to inquire about many things. Naturally, it begins with our every day thoughts and reactions to the people, things and events in our environment. Our reactions until now have been rooted in the many dramas we have created for ourselves over a long, long time. Our reactions will change as we develop the ability to see beyond our inner dramas.

It is a great gift to be coming into a condition with the witness where we can observe our thoughts and feelings as objects playing outside our sense of self. The ability to view external objects and events with a sense of independence will also make a big difference. Then we can question our mental and emotional processes about all of it, without having the extra baggage of feeling that it is somehow us. We can see our dramas for what they are – just stories that we have invented subconsciously to carry us through life.

But are they true stories? If we ask this lovingly when they begin to play, with a desire to know, in the stillness of our abiding witness, we will know the truth. Then what is not true will gradually peel off, or dissolve. When this process becomes a central part of our experience, it is a huge liberation. It is the point where we truly begin to discriminate – making informed choices about what is real in our life, and what is not. In this situation, we will find for the first time that we are able to consciously reverse habitual identifications we have harbored for life.

Prior to the witness, we have been inclined to react in ways that are vested (identified) in our thought patterns and the associated emotional entanglements. The common term is *mental baggage* – all the stories and dramas we carry around with us. In fact, these patterns and entanglements are nothing but habits of the mind, which is a machine whose function is only to produce thoughts based on previous causes and effects. As long as we regard our thoughts and feelings to be us, and our dramas to be real, we will be caught on the wheel of causes and effects.

The primary purpose of self-inquiry is to lead us beyond the knee-jerk reactions associated with this unending series of causes and effects, replacing them with the unaffected observer, the witness. Doing this by rational thinking alone is very difficult, so we bring in the witness with the easy procedure daily deep meditation. This adds the necessary additional dimension of awareness that is beyond time and space, making effective self-inquiry possible.

When we are having negative thoughts, whether they are coming from inside, without any visible external stimulation, or coming in response to external stimuli, we can observe them, and inquire as to their reality. If the thoughts we are having are not in our best interest, we can release them into stillness and not act on them. It is a choice we have. Likewise, if we are receiving external stimuli in the form of communications or events that seem threatening to us, we can inquire as to the reality of the threat. But not if there is obvious danger. In that case, we do what is necessary to protect ourselves.

If someone is taking an action that creates negative thoughts in us, we can inquire about the reality of our thoughts, and choose to release our reaction. We also have the option to *reverse* our reaction. Let's suppose someone says to us, "I hate you!" This may create feelings of anger or inferiority in us. It is not for us to try and change the expression of another as much as it is for us to change our own perception and reaction. This is important.

We cannot change everything in our environment by direct means. However, with the presence of the witness, our perception of everything in our environment can be changed by simple inquiry, release or reversal. What we will find is that, to the degree we are able to change within ourselves, our surrounding environment will be gradually changing also. This is because our perception of our surroundings, including other people, has a direct effect on the quality they will reflect, not only toward us, but toward everyone. If a mean person feels that they are loved unconditionally, a result of our own internal self-inquiry, then it is likely they will be much less mean to everyone. But it is not for us to take responsibility for their conduct, or take on their baggage. It is our responsibility to attend to our own perceptions, thought process, and reactions. This is what self-inquiry of the every day variety is about.

Obviously, if circumstances require immediate action on our part to preserve life and limb, or even a reasonable degree of comfort and convenience, we take that action as necessary. Self-inquiry is not necessarily the best course of action when a truck in bearing down on us. We get out of the way! Then, afterward, we can inquire about the strong thoughts and feelings we may be having then, and release or reverse them.

Our habitual and irrational thought pattern may say, "See, I am worthless, and that truck nearly running me over proves it. Next time it will get me for sure. I was lucky this time."

If we inquire about that, we can just let it go into our stillness, and go on to the next thing in our life, making a note to cross at the intersection next time instead of in the middle of the block. Or, if the negative thought pattern continues, we can ask, "*Is it true that I am worthless? And if so, why?*" The mind may offer an involved rationale for its conclusion that we are worthless, or it may be a mystery as to why we are experiencing such thoughts. Either way, we can witness that process in stillness.

<u>We don't have to engage in a thought process if it is not in our best interest to do so. We can release an untrue thought, or take the opposite thought if we choose.</u>

This is not difficult to do if our inner witness is present. It is the essence of discrimination based in relational self-inquiry. We can choose. *Neti neti* – not this, not this.

So, if our mind is telling us that we are worthless, we don't have to argue with that. We can recognize that it is just a thought, an object in our awareness, and no more true than the thought that we are very worthy. So we can choose to be worthy, rather than worthless. If the mind habitually keeps saying "You are worthless," we can choose to release that thought every single time it comes up. In time, it will lose its power. We don't fight with our negative thoughts, this only strengthens and perpetuates them. Self-inquiry is not about opposing anything. It is only about questioning the reality of our experience, and letting go. In the resulting stillness, we can favor the reversal of the negative thought if we choose.

There is no need for extra analysis, which tends only to build castles in the air, though we need not be concerned much about that if the witness is present. If we build a castle in the air, it can be dissolved just as easily.

Detailed mental analysis can be great fun with the witness in residence, because, when we are truly awake, we do not become identified with our mental structures as we did before. We may become playful with our thought forms. They become quite transparent, and can be whisked away with a simple release into stillness once they have served their purpose. No castle in the air can survive long when seen from the perspective of the witness. If the castle stays there, and keeps getting bigger, this is a sign of non-relational self-inquiry. We will be wise to let it go, and make sure to be continuing our daily deep meditation practice.

The thoughts we give our attention to will be sustained and grow stronger within us. The thoughts we consistently release, because they do not represent the truth of who we are or what we want, will gradually have less influence over us. True self-inquiry is a state of constant release in stillness, which occurs when we reach the dispassion stage of mind discussed in the last chapter.

It is our own energy that feeds the dramas we choose to engage in. Our desire and the choices we make in stillness each day about our own thoughts and feelings determine our path more so than anything else we encounter in life.

The variations on this process are endless, but the basic mechanics are always the same. We observe our thoughts and let them go. We can choose a new direction by easily favoring the new direction over the undesired one. It is a reversal of ingrained patterns in us which we can participate in directly in stillness. Over time, we can release our old negative habits in favor of creating more productive and harmonious ones. Our energies can be redirected to a higher purpose. In this way, abiding inner silence and the rise of divine flow in us can transform our life, and the lives of those around us as well.

Much of this will be automatic as our witness increases in presence. We will naturally see what is true and what is not, and choose our course more wisely than we did before. Feelings like self-condemnation, guilt, jealousy and pride are gradually replaced with feelings of peace, energy, creativity, optimism and love. In short, contraction and unhappiness are replaced with expansion and happiness. The unreal gives way to the real. This is how the truth sets us free.

Over time, our choosing of the higher road in our perceptions, thoughts and feelings becomes automatic, and the habit of negative interpretation (the inner drama) becomes less and less. There will come a time when the only thoughts and feelings we have will be the ones that are suited for the most positive outcome in every situation we encounter in life. Such is the power of the witness and self-inquiry in every day living.

Self-Inquiry for Ultimate Truth

It is human nature to be inquiring about the ultimate truth of existence. We all do it to one degree or other long before we have even begun spiritual practices in this life. And we will inquire even more about it as our practices go forward and mature.

We have an insatiable urge to know who we are and what we are doing here on this earth. It is wired into every human being. All seeking that we do in life, whether for knowledge, fame, or fortune, is ultimately about finding our place in the grand scheme of things.

The irony in this is that we are far greater than any knowledge, fame, or fortune we can possibly gather in this life. And at the same time we are much less, for our true nature is that which is eternal and unbounded, behind and beyond all that occurs on this earth. The least (our awareness) is the greatest, and the greatest (this world) is the least.

The role of self-inquiry in knowing the ultimate truth of existence is very simple – or *realizing* it, as is often said. All we must do is release our perceptions, thoughts and feelings, and what is left is ultimate truth. *That* which underlies all that exists.

Of course, it is easier said than done, because realizing ultimate truth means dissolving every mental and emotional habit we have deeply ingrained in us. If it seems like a high price to pay for realization, it will only be if we are premature in the pursuit. By premature, we mean charging ahead with non-relational self-inquiry without the witness. Without the evolving presence of the witness, self-inquiry of this nature can lead to confusion and conflict in life. It can result in the cessation of all other practices and a loss of interest in fulfilling daily responsibilities.

On the other hand, if the witness is present and becoming gradually more prevalent in our life through daily deep meditation and other sitting practices, then self-inquiry for ultimate truth will become relational, and not a major disruption in our life. This is natural self-inquiry arising about <u>all</u> thoughts, feelings and experiences, both negative and positive. Even our mundane and neutral thoughts are questioned. For the practitioner of relational self-inquiry, the process becomes joyful and never-ending, like a game or a dance. If it is fun, we will know it is relational.

The nature of relational self-inquiry for ultimate truth is such that every thought, feeling and experience is met with the silent impulse, "*Who is experiencing this?*" even as life goes on in all of its ordinary ways. There is no strain or fuss about it. It is very easy and natural.

The inevitable answer to the question is, "I am experiencing this."

Then, what naturally follows is, "*Who am I?*"

There can be many descriptions of who "*I*" is.

"I am Bob or Betty."

"I am this body."

"I am these thoughts."

"I am the one who is here."

Each of these is inquired about in turn, until the last vestige of objectivity has been dissolved, and only the subject remains – the ultimate truth. Even the idea of "*I*" is inquired upon and fades in time, because "*I*" is individuation, and that which is behind all experience is not individual. It is only "*AM*." We could say it is consciousness itself, but we cannot know for sure, because consciousness can only be known in relation to something else. That is why some call the ultimate truth behind life *emptiness*, *nothingness*, *void*, and so on. As we have been saying, in vedanta and yoga, it is simply called *That*.

Those who have the experience of ultimate truth may describe it after-the-fact as having been somewhere – awake, not asleep, being aware, but not of any thought or object. Blissful sensations, boundlessness and a sense of timelessness are often associated with this experience. Perhaps this is why the yogis call it *sat-chit-ananda*, which means *eternal bliss consciousness*. Such experiences, described afterward, are not uncommon for those who engage in deep meditation.

Those who are purists in self-inquiry may deny the existence of any experience at all. This is actually true while one is in the condition of ultimate truth (pure consciousness) where no machinery of experience is operating. Yet, it can be described afterward. So who can say? Experience, or the lack of it, will always be relative to the observer, the mechanics of perception, and the relationship of objects to the subject/witness. The purist would reply that there are no objects, no mechanics of perception, and no afterward, only the eternal condition of truth itself right now – the never-born and never-dying.

As we advance, the inquiry for dissolving our identification with objects will continue even as we go on interacting in time and space ... or seem to be interacting. It is a riddle. "To be, or not to be? That is the question."

One thing that we do know – the witness does coexist with our experience of the world, and enables us to engage in relational self-inquiry. So the riddle is not unsolvable. With deep meditation, the rise of the witness, and self-inquiry, we are able to bootstrap our way to the eternal infinite, the shining void that we come to know as our *Self*.

Most of us who are engaged in self-inquiry would like to have it both ways – to be in the world but not of the world. It is a natural desire, and suitable to keep us on the path. This is the goal of all spiritual practice – to find freedom from suffering, even while still in the body. More than that – to find happiness and meaning in life.

Purists in self-inquiry seek to remain beyond the suffering of the world. As part of this, they may also seek to remain beyond happiness and any meaning that might be found in earthly life. The purist may not acknowledge the expressions of divine love that accompany human enlightenment. The enlightened cannot help themselves, and often go to great lengths in expressing divine love to teach others how to be free themselves. Even so, such spontaneous acts may be regarded by the purist as froth upon the ocean of emptiness. And, indeed, they are just that.

What remains when the truth is fully realized are desireless desires and actless acts of love and kindness. In AYP we call it *stillness in action*, or *outpouring divine love*.

The task of self-inquiry is not to end thinking, feeling and action, but to become *That* which is beyond thinking, feeling and action. In doing so, thinking, feeling and action will go on, but the doer is nowhere to be found. For that *One* is beyond all doing. What remains is *divine doing*.

On the practical level, this end state can be cultivated with a full range of yoga practices, beginning with daily deep meditation. Self-inquiry then comes along quite naturally.

If self-inquiry is forced before the witness has dawned, life will be strained and confused, and results will be slow in coming. If the witness is present, self-inquiry will be there on the practical level of living in a way that allows us to continue our involvement in daily activities without constantly questioning our reasons for being engaged in living. The reasons will become clear enough as the witness evolves within us and we gradually come to realize who we are and what we are doing here.

Then, questions like *"Who is writing this book?"* or *"Who is reading this book?"* will be answered in stillness, and we will just go on. If we easily favor the question in our stillness, the answer will be there. And we will know that it is stillness who is writing, and it is stillness who is reading.

Pitfalls of the Mind

The mind is a marvelous machine, capable of performing many great feats of analysis, deduction and discovery. It is also the mind that enables us to create the sense of *"I"* within us. "I am Mary." "I am this body." "I am this mind." "I was born, I am living, and someday I will die."

The purpose of self-inquiry is to use the mind to question and transcend these assumptions that are associated with "I am…"

When combined with the presence of the witness resulting from daily deep meditation, self-inquiry reveals that we are not our name, our form, or even our sense of *"I."* What we are is the stillness behind and within all that is being projected. So, the first pitfall of the mind is *identification*. That is, the identification of our awareness with all the things that are projected out into time and space.

Indeed, identification may be the only pitfall of the mind. The mind has a tendency to ramble on about our life experiences, whether they be in the past, present or future. And the mind will paint it as positive or negative, according to our mood. It is always about one thing – the mind wrapping us up in something.

Is this the mind's fault? Is there something inherently dysfunctional about the human mind? Or is it something else? After all, the mind is only a machine. Do we blame the automobile when it skids off the road into a tree? Do we blame the hammer when it hits our thumb? Well, maybe some of us do. And perhaps that is a symptom of the underlying problem. If the driver will not take responsibility for the automobile, and the carpenter will not take responsibility for the hammer, then who will? Likewise, if the inhabitant of the mind will not take responsibility for its actions, who will?

Who is the inhabitant of the mind? It is we who are aware, to whatever degree we are aware. The less aware the inhabitant of the mind is, the less likely will the mind be performing as it is designed to, as a servant. Then the mind will be more likely to be operating as a sorcerer's apprentice, feigning leadership and casting a web of confusion over life. Where there is a vacuum of awareness (the witness not present much) the mind will rush to fill the void with the only thing it can fill it with – lots of thoughts and false perceptions, which are in turn translated to be, "I am these objects of perception..." rather than, "I am the subject, the eternal awareness interpenetrating all these objects..."

So, the first step in helping the mind get back to its rightful purpose is to make sure the inhabitant of the mind will be present and fully awake. This is the witness, and we know the prescription by now – daily deep meditation. With the inhabitant of the mind moving in and taking the reins, there will be steady improvement in the operation of the mind. As the clamp of identification is loosened, the functioning of the mind will improve all the way around.

But the full integration of inner silence with the mind is not an overnight affair. It takes time. Even with the natural emergence of desire to engage in self-inquiry, there is still a long road to travel to full enlightenment. Along the road there are some particular pitfalls of the mind that may jeopardize our spiritual progress. These are the kinds of pitfalls we'd like to address here, because they can have a bearing on our ability to sustain practices and continued progress on our path:

- Infatuation with or fear of spiritual experiences.
- Over-analyzing and over-philosophizing.
- Overdoing self-inquiry or other yoga practices.
- The illusion of attainment, or of having "arrived."
- Denial of the need to engage in practices.
- The non-duality trap – denying the world.

Such pitfalls of the mind can hamper a spiritual aspirant at any stage along the path. Advanced practitioners are equally susceptible to be drawn off course, perhaps more-so when visited by dramatic experiences of the vastness of pure bliss consciousness, ecstatic bliss, and miraculous powers of one sort or other. These kinds of experiences can rock the mind if inner silence (the witness) has not yet been cultivated to a sufficient level of maturity in the nervous system, enabling the practitioner to take advanced spiritual experiences in stride.

So, whether we are just starting out on our path, or are quite far along, cultivating the witness will be the best insurance we can have to guard against the pitfalls of the mind.

Infatuation or Fear about Experiences

Spiritual experiences come in many forms and, if we are utilizing effective yoga practices, such experiences will always be associated with purification and opening occurring within us. When experiences come, we will be inclined to think something about them. How we regard them will be a function of our understanding of the processes of yoga and the degree of presence of inner witness we have.

When experience is dramatic, when we are overcome with a large energy flow or a vision of our vastness and unity with all things, then we may become identified with the experience. A kind of infatuation can happen then, or even some fear about what we have gotten ourselves into, especially if the internal energy flow becomes excessive, which can lead to a variety of physical and psychological symptoms – also referred to as *kundalini symptoms*.

If we have been approaching our practice from the point of view of our limited self, rather than from the point of view of the witness, we may become infatuated in a way that is similar to romantic infatuation. All infatuations do pass, of course, and in the meantime, we will be wise to favor our practice over the experience. When we are engaged in sitting practices, we can just easily favor the practice we are doing over visions or energy experiences that are coming. If we are in our daily activity, then we can just carry on with our work, whatever it may be.

If experiences overwhelm us to the point where we become fearful that we may be losing control of our life, then it can be helpful to stay engaged in life, particularly in activities that are *grounding*. These are physical activities, and activities that are about helping others. At the same time we can temporarily reduce the kinds of activities that stimulate spiritual energy flows, such as attending spiritual gatherings and too much spiritual practice. We have mentioned earlier that this temporary ramping down of spiritual stimulation is called *self-pacing*. Such regulation is a primary consideration in the AYP approach, where an integration of powerful practices is being utilized in a self-directed manner.

Infatuation will pass and fear will subside as inner purification advances and we find a natural integration of the divine within us in every day living. This is why it is best to carry on with our life, no matter what our spiritual experiences may be. Ultimately, enlightenment is about marrying the spectacular with the ordinary. What remains is spectacular ordinariness.

Over-Analyzing and Over-Philosophizing

Whether we are having spiritual experiences or not, constant analysis and philosophizing about our condition (past, present, or future), will not be of much benefit. In fact, this tendency is one of the most common forms of non-relational self-inquiry.

When an experience comes up, whether it be physical, mental, or emotional, we will have a tendency to analyze it. It will be good to understand that taking this to the point of obsession is a common pitfall of the mind.

This doesn't mean we do not analyze or seek confirmation of our path in the scriptures and philosophies that have been written over the centuries. But if we make analysis or philosophy the object of our path, we will be veering off on a tangent that can undermine our commitment to yoga practices and relational self-inquiry. When analysis and philosophy creep up to the point where they become ends in themselves, then we have entered into the realm of building castles in the air, which is non-relational and not effective spiritual practice.

In that case, we can just observe and let go of the excessive analysis in favor of cultivating the witness in our sitting practices, and going out and living our life fully.

Overdoing Self-Inquiry or other Yoga Practices

A common pitfall of the mind is found in the idea that if a little of a particular practice is bringing us some results, then a lot more of it will bring even more results.

For example, if we have asked ourselves, "*Who am I?*" and a flash of inspiration comes, we might conclude that we should be asking ourselves "*Who am I?*" twenty-four hours per day, seven days per week.

Likewise, if we have been engaging in daily deep meditation twice each day for twenty minutes (a balanced practice), and find a noticeable presence of the inner witness coming up, then we might conclude that meditating much longer and more often will be better.

In either case (non-stop self-inquiry or non-stop deep meditation), we will be stepping into a mental pitfall that can actually slow our spiritual progress. Overdoing practices will only produce excessive purification and strain that will limit our ability to practice effectively until balance has returned.

While some teachers preach the possibility of instant enlightenment, that all we are is here and now, it does in fact take some time to open up the nervous system to our greater possibilities within. It is a process, which can be accelerated in particular ways, but not on a flight of fancy that more is always going to be better. The path to enlightenment involves a process that takes time, no matter what methods we are following, and there are few shortcuts that can bypass the need for self-pacing in practices.

Rome was not built in a day; and neither is the process of *human spiritual transformation* completed in a day. If we are steadfast in applying tried and true methods over time, the result will be there. The journey to enlightenment is a marathon, not a sprint.

The Illusion of Attainment or of Having Arrived

Enlightenment, the direct realization of who we are, is unassuming and does not proclaim itself, except by compassionate assistance offered for the benefit of everyone. Conversely, where there is the assumption of attainment or of having arrived, actions can be distorted accordingly, leading to a rigid teaching, proselytizing, sectarianism, and a shift in focus from spiritual practices to the one who has supposedly arrived. It is a pitfall of the mind commonly found on either the side of the teacher, the student, or both.

When consciousness is identified with the mind, there will be a great need to proclaim victory over the forces of ignorance. This breeds more ignorance, of course. There can be no enlightenment proclaimed on the level of the mind. The functioning of the mind can only be seen as a symptom of the illumination which comes from within, or the lack of it. We may conclude that an inner flow is occurring or not, but we can never proclaim with accuracy that we have arrived, for that is beyond the province of the mind.

By definition, both the cause and the destination of true self-inquiry are beyond the mind, in the abiding inner witness, which never assumes or proclaims anything. It just is.

When there is some proclaiming going on, it is wise to ask, *"Who is proclaiming?"* and then let go in stillness.

Denying Practices

There are rare cases of individuals who reach what seems to be an enlightened state in this life with little or no effort in spiritual practices. It is natural for such individuals to promote the idea of enlightenment requiring no practices from their unique point of view. They routinely will say, "There is nothing to do. You are there already."

It is like the New Yorker who mysteriously wakes up in Los Angeles one day, not knowing how he got there, and then calling all his friends in New York to tell them they can do the same. If only…

This kind of teaching is flawed, to say the least. While the destination may be true, the means will be lacking for nearly everyone. So, when a teacher tells us that we need do nothing to reach enlightenment, and we do not find ourselves there in that instant, then it will be wise to review additional means that are available. In this case the conclusion of the enlightened one is a mental pitfall (yes, they do have them), and to follow such a teaching to the exclusion of everything else is a mental pitfall in the student.

A common symptom of the illusion of having arrived can be a loss of recognition of the value of spiritual practices. It is one of the greatest risks for advanced practitioners – falling into the belief that our journey to realization is done. The next thought the mind will produce is, "I don't have to practice any more." And wherever we are on the path at that point, that is more or less where we will stay until we wake up enough to realize that our spiritual progress never ends, and therefore the need for spiritual practice will never end either. Practices may change according to our ongoing purification and opening, but the need for them will never end.

The reason is because there is no such thing as individual enlightenment in the ultimate sense. As we are approaching individual enlightenment, we know ourselves to be all that is around us. Then the condition of consciousness of all who are around us is seen to be our condition. So we will not be fully enlightened until everyone is enlightened. This is why so-called enlightened people continue to work for the benefit of all. Their liberation will not be fulfilled until everyone's is. And neither shall ours. There is much joy and fulfillment to be found along the way, as long as we continue with our practices, yielding ever-increasing expansion to the infinite!

The Non-Duality Trap – Denying the World

Sages may tell us that the world is not real, but a projection occurring via our senses and the perception of objects through the identification of our awareness. On the other hand, it has been said that perception is 100% of reality, and this is also true. Our reality is what we perceive it to be. But the sage will say that it is all illusion, and that if we deconstruct the machinery of identification of our awareness with our perceptions, we will find that there is nothing here at all.

Well, true. We learned it in high school quantum physics. But is this a useful view of our world? Can we continue to function with such a view when taken on the level of the intellect alone? Not likely.

While the logic of non-duality is impeccable, the assumption that it can be realized instantly by everyone is incorrect. Those teachers who disregard the perceptions of others (100% of *their* reality) and refuse to meet them where they are will fail to help them. In fact, damage can be done by encouraging students to reach far beyond where they are without offering intermediate steps.

We know that if we try to run before we have learned to crawl and walk, we will land flat on our face and may find ourselves in serious trouble with our motivation and ability to function in the world. For the vast majority of practitioners of self-inquiry, laboring to deny the existence of the world is destructive. While we can certainly find inspiration in the concept of *Oneness without second*, to attempt to live that in the mind is a huge pitfall. This is because *Oneness* (non-duality) is not of the mind. As soon as we try and live it there, we will find much of our life to be meaningless, experiencing a false rejection of every day living, and this is very unhealthy. This is non-relational self-inquiry at its worst.

The paradox in this is that the experience of *Oneness* is highly meaningful in all aspects of life, and is the source of all love and sharing in unity. The non-dual condition is an experience of unity, of radiant love and joining, not an experience of separation – not a denial of the world at all.

If we are doing self-inquiry with the presence of the witness, we will not fall into the trap of denying *life as it is*. Instead we will find ourselves coming more and more into the condition of *becoming* life as it is, which can also be described as being in the world but not of the world. This is real *Oneness*, real non-duality. Not the divisive non-relational kind of self-inquiry that can lead to years of struggle and misery. There is a better way of affirming the sacred proclamation of the sages that "All are *One*."

Self-Inquiry and the Limbs of Yoga

Self-inquiry is found in all systems of spiritual development. Wherever there is discrimination on the spiritual path, there will be self-inquiry. Whether it is relational self-inquiry or not is another matter, and that is the key question. Is the witness present when we are inquiring?

Some systems of spiritual development are philosophical by nature and teachers may subscribe to self-inquiry as a stand-alone practice in order to adhere to the strict tenets of the philosophy. The philosophical system of *Vedanta* is one of these, and its strong stance on the non-dual (advaita) nature of existence, and the non-existence of the world, may leave the practitioner with little choice but to declare the truth of non-duality, whether it is being experienced or not ... or just walk away muttering.

Vedanta means the *end of the Veda* (the end of knowledge). It relies on Indian scriptures such as the *Upanishads* and *Brahma Sutras* to make its case for the non-duality of existence. The case is philosophically sound, if not easily realized outright by the average student. Vedanta also relies on the *Bhagavad Gita* to support its assertion that existence is non-dual in its nature, and therefore the world will be known to be unreal even when we are fully engaged in worldly activities. Fair enough.

Interestingly, the system and philosophy of spiritual development known as *Yoga* finds validation in these same ancient scriptures, even though yoga is often regarded as a *dual* rather than *non-dual* approach. Yoga also subscribes to and has its origin in the *Yoga Sutras of Patanjali*, which prescribe a range of practices designed to bring about the very condition of non-duality (*Oneness*) held by vedanta as the ultimate truth.

The remaining systems of Indian philosophy and spiritual development are about equally split with regard to being considered dual or non-dual in their approach. There are six systems in all, give or take, depending on who is doing the counting. All of these systems recognize the unified nature of existence, just as high school quantum physics does nowadays.

This raises a question: If all of the systems recognize the non-dual nature of existence, then which one is the right one in its approach?

The answer is, it depends what you are looking for. What is not often suggested is that all of the systems, and their methods, can be applied <u>together</u> for maximum effect. If the boundaries between them are dissolved, then the best of all worlds can be realized – *Oneness*. This will not be easy for those with a sectarian streak, which is a paradox for those who may consider themselves to be staunch non-dualists. How can *anything* be separated from that point of view?

Yoga does not suffer from such conflicts, and happily embraces all philosophies and systems of spiritual practice that lead to the best results. At least the most effective yoga systems do.

Patanjali was so complete in laying out his famous *Eight Limbs of Yoga* that yoga philosophy is able to accommodate many angles of approach for cultivating the process of human spiritual transformation. He may not have intended it that way, but his all-inclusive model, reflecting the full range of capabilities for spiritual transformation found in the human nervous system, has turned out to be compatible with multiple strategies and systems. The eight limbs form a good checklist for considering the completeness of any system of spiritual practice.

Patanjali's eight limbs of yoga include:

- **Yama** (*restraints* – non-violence, truthfulness, non-stealing, preservation and cultivation of sexual energy, and non-covetousness)
- **Niyama** (*observances* – purity, contentment, spiritual intensity, study of spiritual knowledge and *Self*, and active surrender to the divine)
- **Asana** (postures and physical maneuvers)
- **Pranayama** (breathing techniques)
- **Pratyahara** (introversion of the senses)
- **Dharana** (systematic attention on an object)
- **Dhyana** (meditation – systematic dissolving of the object)
- **Samadhi** (absorption in pure consciousness)

There is an additional category of practice called **Samyama**, which integrates the last three limbs of yoga together – dharana, dhyana and samadhi. The mechanics of samyama are closely related to the performance of relational self-inquiry, as is further discussed below.

Self-inquiry is included in the Niyamas (observances) in the form of *study of spiritual knowledge and Self*, and is also woven throughout all of the eight limbs in the form of *discrimination*, where particular modes of practice are easily favored over the many forms of experience that can arise. Taken together as a systematic integration, the methods of yoga bring realization of the same truth of non-dual *Oneness* that is expounded in vedanta. It is accomplished by promoting a gradual process of purification and opening within the human nervous system, leading to its highest expressions of abiding inner silence, ecstatic bliss, and the unity of outpouring divine love.

Of course, regardless of its logic, such a multi-pronged *cause and effect* approach might make a devout non-dualist cringe. But, as has been discussed earlier, if real (relational) self-inquiry is going to be happening, cultivation of the inner witness via deep meditation, as a minimum, will be a prudent course. In the language of the eight limbs of yoga, the witness in daily activity is abiding samadhi (pure consciousness). There are many names for it. We will know the witness when we see it, and are it. A rose is still a rose by any other name.

Just as there are those with a fixed view of vedanta, there are people within yoga who subscribe to a singular practice, or other narrow approaches to the exclusion of the rest of yoga, and everything else. It is easy to get stuck in a mode of little progress when taking a narrow view in yoga, vedanta, or any approach to spiritual realization. It takes a flexible integration of methods to penetrate the veil of ideas, emotions and perceived materiality in front of us, to realize the eternal luminous reality underlying it all, which is our true *Self.* Just as a broad view of the systems of Indian philosophy can be beneficial, so too will a broad application of the methods of yoga be more likely to bring results than a narrowly focused view.

This is consistent with the goal of vedanta – the realization of the non-dual nature of existence. With an ongoing intent to drop our imaginary boundaries both in perceptions and in practices, and a willingness to utilize the full range of tools that are available to aid in this, then we will be on our way. It will only be a matter of determining what methods to apply, and in which order. It will be largely a matter of personal preference, and a logical application of causes and effects to find out what works best for us.

Devotion and Self-Inquiry

No matter what our spiritual path may be, it will have its origin and ongoing sustenance in our desire. It is our longing for truth and a willingness to act upon our longing that is the root cause of everything else that occurs on our path.

It has been said that a prerequisite to enlightenment is the end of all desire. This is not entirely true. Without desire there can be no path, and no practice of any kind. Even if we deny the need for practice in favor of stand-alone self-inquiry, a desire for truth will still be necessary to keep us going in that.

Desire in relation to the spiritual path is often misunderstood. As we come into a direct realization of the truth of what we are, it is true that our desire for the ephemeral things of this world will become less. A reduction in this kind of desire is *effect* rather than cause – a tail on the dog of rising realization. Even as our worldly desire may become less, our spiritual desire will be increasing in kind. Exponentially, some might say. So enlightenment is not about ending desire. It is about shifting it naturally to higher truth, until all desire is dissolved in the reality of *Oneness*, which is experienced as an unending outpouring of divine love. Then our desire has become synonymous with divine desire, and continues on...

An intentional desire for the realization of truth is not only useful, it is essential. When desire is directed toward a high ideal, and is sustained, it is called *devotion*. In the language of yoga, this is called *bhakti*.

Besides the obvious motivational power of devotion inspiring us to take action on our path toward realization, there is an *innate power of transformation* in devotion that directly stimulates inner purification and opening, independent of any other action taken on our part. In other words, devotion alone has the power to open us to the truth, assuming the ideal of our devotion reaches beyond where we are today. This natural feature of devotion is why it is the most prevalent spiritual practice in all of the world's religions. Devotion to a high spiritual ideal (divine personage, icon, condition or concept) is at the core of all spiritual progress, whether additional methods are being applied or not.

Of course, as soon as we begin integrating additional effective methods with our spiritual desire, our rate of transformation to realization will be accelerating. In fact, it is devotion that leads us to all additional means. Devotion increases the effectiveness of all additional means we undertake, whether it be deep meditation, self-inquiry, or any other spiritual practice.

So, even if we are highly orthodox in our approach to self-inquiry, denying all other forms of practice, we cannot deny that it is our desire that is carrying us forward, raised to the level of unending devotion (bhakti) to a high ideal. There is something that is leading us to the ultimate freedom of realization of our non-dual nature. That something is devotion, the unifying power of divine love emanating from within our stillness.

Meditation, Samyama and Self-Inquiry

A prerequisite for self-inquiry is inner silence, or the witness. When the witness is present we have relational self-inquiry. And when the witness is lacking to the point where our self-inquiry is merely thoughts interacting with more thoughts, with limited connection between the inquiry and the native awareness which is behind it, then we say the practice is non-relational.

We have discussed the role of deep meditation in cultivating the witness, so the relationship between meditation and self-inquiry on that score is clear. However, there is more we can say about deep meditation as it relates to cultivating a *key ability* in the mind. We can say that in deep meditation we find the procedural seeds for true relational self-inquiry. What is this key ability?

Stated quite simply, in deep meditation we are cultivating inner silence (the witness) in a systematic way by easily favoring an object in the mind over all other thoughts and perceptions. This is done by gently favoring the object whenever we are aware that we have drifted off the object. The object is called a *mantra*, which is the thought of particular sound that is used with a procedure that enables us to systematically bring attention to its core in pure consciousness, beyond all thinking. In the AYP approach, the mantra we use is *I AM*. For more on the procedure of deep meditation, see the additional resources listed on the last page of this book. The procedure for using the mantra is at the heart of deep meditation, and also is at the heart of the rise of the witness in daily life.

The rise of the witness is also at the heart of relational self-inquiry. In fact, we can say that the dawn of the witness is the beginning of self-inquiry. The ability we develop by easily favoring the mantra, which leads to stillness in deep meditation, is the same *key ability* we utilize in easily favoring the witness in self-inquiry.

As we continue to meditate on a twice daily basis, we are conditioning the mind to reside in stillness as an automatic habit, even in the face of a never-ending avalanche of thoughts, feelings, perceptions, and actions we are engaged in. Developing this habit of being in stillness, even as we are active in the world, is also the essential objective and desired outcome of self-inquiry. Once we have cultivated the witness in this manner, we have also developed the *key ability* necessary for self-inquiry, which is being able to allow thoughts and perceptions to pass by in favor of stillness. We don't have to cling to them anymore, or the associated inner dramas we have created in the past, for we have found our sense of self, our home, in something more pleasing, more lasting, and more present. Pure consciousness – our own *Self.*

Samyama is a logical stepping stone once we have become established in deep meditation and find abiding inner silence coming up. It is a systematic means for developing the ability to infuse every aspect of our thinking and action with the quality of the witness. In deep meditation we refine the object (mantra) and dissolve it in stillness, thus cultivating witness. In samyama we systematically bring stillness out into all of the objects in our life and dissolve them in that way. Deep meditation works from the outside in. Samyama works from the inside out.

Samyama is dissolving the illusion of the material world by bringing inner silence outward via our intentions into our every day actions. Just as for self-inquiry, some degree of inner silence (witness) is a necessary prerequisite for samyama.

As our ability to *flow outward as stillness* develops naturally in daily life, aided greatly by regular samyama practice, we find increasing translucence in the world, and we experience through direct perception that we are living as *stillness in action.* Then we come to see the world for what it is, an infinite field of joyful emptiness in motion.

Samyama and self-inquiry are closely related, as both are about the same thing – cultivating the habit of operating within stillness. As our experience becomes more pervasive (first by cultivation of the static witness in deep meditation, and then by cultivation of the dynamic witness in samyama), our self-inquiry becomes greatly enhanced at the same time, simply by observing what is before us through direct perception. Then it becomes easy to let go of thoughts and perceptions that previously had hold over us through the process of identification of awareness with perceptions of external phenomena.

What we find with the advancement of our witness from static to dynamic is the ability to inquire relationally from within every object we encounter, because we have become every object by direct experience. Our *"I"* sense has both gone beyond objects and begun to inhabit objects at the same time. It is one of those divine paradoxes.

Deep meditation and samyama add a huge dimension of effectiveness to our self-inquiry. In fact, these practices make self-inquiry inevitable, for the simple reason that *seeing is believing*. We could say that advanced relational self-inquiry is a form of samyama, where we are automatically releasing into stillness all of our thoughts, feelings and perceptions of the external world. When we see what the nature of existence is, we are easily able to discriminate what is true from what is not without hesitation. Self-inquiry becomes an instant and automatic part of our every day navigation through life, and we move quickly onward from discrimination into dispassion, outpouring divine love and unity. Then we are doing everything while doing nothing!

Kundalini and Self-Inquiry

The word *kundalini* and the phenomena it describes have received much fanfare and notoriety. If we are developing a serious approach to self-inquiry, even when recognizing the essential roles of our devotion, deep meditation and samyama, we may be tempted to ignore the thing called *kundalini,* because it is so deeply associated with the body. Of all the aspects of yoga, kundalini is the part that seems to be most deeply rooted in the duality of existence, and therefore of least interest to someone who is seeking to realize the highest truth.

Nothing could be further from the truth.

Kundalini is about the energetic development of our subtle neurobiology, giving rise to the direct perception of radiant *Oneness* in our environment. While even this perception is ultimately transcended, it is a necessary stepping stone that all who are on the path will take. Even if the process of kundalini is ignored, the aspirant will still experience it as part of the journey to realization. If the nature of kundalini and its various symptoms are not understood, it can lead to delays in our development, because the risk of falling into unknowing distraction with our inner energies will be much higher.

Like self-inquiry, a smooth and natural unfoldment of kundalini can be facilitated by developing a good foundation of inner silence (the witness) early on. Once that has been done via deep meditation, then other methods can be applied to assure a safe and progressive cultivation of kundalini, the ecstatic energetic side of our nature that leads first to ecstatic energy flowing, and later on to direct perception of the transcendent shining radiance that is within us and everywhere in our environment .

This is important, because full realization will not occur until <u>both</u> inner silence and ecstatic conductivity have matured and joined within us. This is the essential neurobiology of enlightenment found wherever human spiritual transformation is occurring, no matter what means are being utilized, including self-inquiry.

Self-inquiry will not find its fruition until all of the associated inner neurobiological processes have reached their maturation and fulfillment. If we do not attend to them in a systematic manner, they will occur anyway, possibly in a chaotic way. If we have a choice (and we do), then a systematic approach will be preferred by most of us over an approach leading through chaos. Not only that – systematic is *much faster* than chaotic, so it is an easy choice. If we want to be stubborn about it and ignore the inevitable stages of inner transformation in favor of a fixed philosophical approach, then we will pay the price in both progress and comfort.

Those who are truly able to *let go* will notice the energetic processes occurring within them, and do what is necessary to optimize them for a speedy and safe journey into realization. Those who hang on to a fixed view will face the ironic situation of hanging on to letting go, to the exclusion of everything else, including the actual process of human spiritual transformation that is occurring.

Kundalini is a vast subject, which can fill volumes. We will not overdo it here. Nor do we overdo it anywhere in the AYP writings. It is an aspect of the whole of our realization that should be taken into account, and is covered as necessary to support the over all journey. We will know it when we see it, and be much better prepared to move ahead rather than become stalled in energy distractions. Relational self-inquiry can be used to favor progress in stillness over the temptations of infatuation with the inevitable ecstatic energy experiences that will happen along the way. We can release them in self-inquiry, just as we can all identifications with experience we may be prone to indulge in.

Yoga addresses the energetic side of our development through pranayama (breathing techniques), asanas (postures), mudras and bandhas (inner physical maneuvers), and tantric methods (the management of sexual energy in particular). All of these are easily incorporated into our sitting practices and the normal conduct of our daily life, in the same way that self-inquiry is naturally incorporated when we find the witness coming up and know that we are ready.

It is all part of the same journey, and no part of it is favored over the other. Each aspect evolves in its own time, and we know that each step is the right one by its natural emergence and observable results. In that sense, all yoga practices are known by their relational resonance with each other, our inner silence, and our every day activities. We will know we are in balance if life is getting better, even as we are moving steadily into a condition of non-duality, which is no condition at all, of course.

Self-inquiry has a direct role to play in the unfoldment of kundalini as it purifies and opens us via the central channel, or spinal nerve, running between our perineum and center brow. It is an aspect of the *key ability* developed in deep meditation, discussed in the last section – simply to allow the kundalini process to occur as it will while naturally releasing our attention in stillness. This helps us to avoid going off into flights of fancy when dramatic kundalini symptoms occur, which they surely shall at some time or other.

It is like all experiences in life. We gradually come to know them all to be waves upon the ocean of our infinite inner silence. The difference between kundalini experiences and the rest of our experiences in life is that kundalini experiences can be dramatic, involving a range of physical symptoms, large surges of inner energy and ecstasy, visions, sounds and other internal sensory perceptions. The emotions can also be affected, sometimes positively and sometimes negatively in the case of excessive energy flows. All of this will have a corresponding effect on our mind, and this is why self-inquiry (relational – in stillness) can be very helpful. We know that it is all just *scenery* we are passing by on the road to realization.

While the scenery is not important in itself, it does have relevance for gaging our speed and comfort on the path. If we are going too fast (too heavy on practices) then the symptoms of purification can become intense, causing us considerable discomfort and/or potential distraction. The process of introversion of sensory perceptions (*pratyahara*) can be moving too fast sometimes. It is important for us to be inquiring about the intensity of our experiences, so we can make adjustments in practices to maintain smooth progress with safety. If we don't do this, we can end up overdoing to the point where we will not be able to practice at all for a while. Then we will have to implement the appropriate *kundalini remedies* and wait until balance is reestablished again before resuming practices (including self-inquiry), which can take valuable time.

We have called this process of gaging the intensity of experiences and scaling our practices accordingly, *self-pacing*. It is an important part of the AYP approach, and is also an aspect of self-inquiry. We always favor the practice over the experience, and scale our practice according to the intensity of the experience, as needed.

The energetic/kundalini side of the process of human spiritual transformation is an aspect that is best not ignored. And neither should it be over-indulged in.

Yama, Niyama and Self-Inquiry

Yama and niyama are the *restraints and observances*, which are generally synonymous with the codes of conduct found in every spiritual tradition – the proverbial *do's and don't's*.

"Thou shalt do this."

"Thou shalt not do that."

But this common definition is an over-simplification, and even a distortion of what yama and niyama really are, and, for that matter, what all spiritual codes of conduct are.

What yama and niyama describe are the behaviors that are inherent in our rising spiritual awareness. With effective spiritual practices in place, these are found to be *effects* more-so than *causes* of spiritual progress.

It has long been believed that conduct constitutes a primary path for promoting human spiritual transformation, and this is why there has been so much emphasis on following rules for centuries in the spiritual traditions. Yet, there are countless examples of people who have devoted their lives to good spiritual conduct and works, only to find at the end that they were little closer to divine realization than they were at the beginning. So something has been missing.

There is certainly practical value in enforcing some standards of conduct in society, particularly in the area of how our actions might harm others. Otherwise there would be lawlessness and mayhem throughout the world. However, placing a singular focus on spiritual conduct is a poor way to promote spiritual progress.

Self-inquiry is also a form of conduct, no matter which form of it we happen to be using – the "every day living" variety, or the "focus on ultimate truth" variety. In fact, all of the restraints and observances rely on *discrimination* (an aspect of self-inquiry) for their performance. In any form of self-inquiry, we are choosing a particular conduct in thought, not just as a practice we do at predetermined times, but eventually as a natural habit in every waking moment. It can only work if it is relational – flying on the wings of our inner witness.

Perhaps over a long period of time, we can elevate a stand-alone self-inquiry practice to the level of an automatic habit. Perhaps we can accomplish this in living strictly by rules of conduct too. But we must ask ourselves if we are developing habits in thought only. Or are we developing habits in stillness? There is a big difference between thinking about letting go of a tendency toward undesired conduct and actually letting go of the tendency. Letting go can only be accomplished in the presence of the witness, and that is relational self-inquiry. Thoughts letting go into more thoughts is non-relational self-inquiry.

A shift from non-relational to relational inquiry happens in yama and niyama as we develop spiritually. So we must ask, are we engaged in spiritual behaviors for the sake of being engaged in spiritual behaviors? Or are we engaged in them because we are moved from within our inner silence to do so? Behavior for the sake of behavior (for the sake of rules) is non-relational, though sometimes necessary to protect us from harm. Behavior for the sake of the divine flow of stillness is relational, and naturally supports the positive flow of evolution everywhere.

This is not to say we do not pursue behaviors we know to be right. The very desire to do so is a sign of rising realization. We may find that this urge occurs more so as we find the witness to be more present in our every day life. It is deep meditation that is actually the fountainhead of spiritual conduct, because it is the primary means for cultivating the witness.

We can, therefore, consider the manifestation of spiritual conduct and the rise of relational self-inquiry to be aspects of the same dynamic in our lives, with both being intertwined with and a direct result of the dawn of the witness.

This underlying principle applies in every area of life, whether we are considering what to do in our career, how to handle our relationships, what to eat, or what yoga practices to undertake. All of these things involve choices, and contain self-inquiry. We'd like to be considering them from the point of view of the witness, rather than by rote rules of conduct.

While some may argue that we have spread self-inquiry out into too many aspects of spiritual practice, it is all for practicality. The uncompromising practitioner of self-inquiry for ultimate truth will release all of this for the sake of the non-dual *One*, which is beyond the external veneer of existence and all of these considerations. Yet, even the absolutist in non-dual self-inquiry must get up in the morning, get dressed, eat, and relate to those who come around. Maybe such a one is beyond the trivial considerations of everyone else who is on the path. But will that be helpful to any but the few who have also transcended the need to navigate through the process of spiritual transformation?

Certainly an end view is important, but it will be the real view only for those who are living it already. For everyone else, effective means are necessary. It is much better to take an airplane from New York to Los Angeles than to try and wish ourselves there.

So, we take self-inquiry for all it is worth on every level, in every nook and cranny of the process of human spiritual transformation. We allow self-inquiry to function fully in concert with the effective methods of integrated yoga practice.

Chapter 4 – The End of Suffering

Before we can consider what constitutes the end of suffering, we will need a practical understanding of what it is.

What is suffering?

It is our identification with pain. And because identification is a function of the mind, suffering will be conjured up by the mind not only in relation to pain experienced in the present, but also in the form of memories from past pain, and the anticipation of future pain. For those who habitually suffer, good health and physical comfort may offer little relief, because the mind can provide an endless supply of past hurts to lament and mountains of worries about the discomforts of the future, none of which exist!

In fact, a person's health, material prospects and external quality of life may have little relationship to how much or how little they suffer, since suffering is the product of identification rooted deep in the mind.

Those who seem to have everything going for them may suffer more than those who may seem to have little. Identification with material wealth and worldly achievements (fortune and fame) can lead to some of the most severe suffering – a dream of life that turns into a nightmare. Why? Because, in that case, we have hitched our wagon to the temporary things of life. No matter how glorious they may seem, they will not last. It is the mistake we make in assuming that we are what we are perceiving. And we pay dearly for that mistake.

Suffering itself is painful, but there is a difference between the pain of suffering and the pain that comes to us from an illness, physical injury or traumatic event. The pain of suffering is imposed by the mind and can be reduced and eventually eliminated through spiritual methods, while the pain of real-time events, may or may not be able to be avoided. In any case, if we are able to release suffering, release identification with what pains us, then the inevitable discomforts and calamities that occur in the ups and downs of life will lose their grip on us also. When our identification with pain has been dissolved, then suffering will be no more.

Who Suffers?

The next time we are in pain, physically or mentally, and feel that we are suffering, we might ask ourselves the question, "*Who is suffering?*"

If we are honest about it, we will find it is our interpretation of the pain that is causing us to perceive ourselves to be suffering. If we are making a value judgment about our pain, we will surely be suffering. We will know we are making a value judgment if we are asking, "*Why me?*" or are placing blame, having anger, or are trying to get others to share in our pain. In all of these reactions we are identified with our pain.

On the other hand, if we see our pain only as pain without coloring it one way or the other, it will still be pain, but there will be no suffering – no judgment about it, no lamentations, no past regrets, no inner drama playing, no fear about it for the future.

When we see someone bearing pain in this way, we tend to call them *spiritual*. They seem to be on a higher plane of consciousness, and the pain of the moment is not touching them in a way that is seen in the mental reaction we call suffering. This does not mean they will not react to the pain with a grimace or by crying out.

Whether we have broken a bone or lost a loved one, we will feel the pain of it, and cry out. Going beyond suffering doesn't mean we will like being in pain. Neither does it mean that we should not do everything we can to remove our pain, and everyone else's. But, whatever may be happening, the scars of suffering will not be with us, not even in the next minute, if we have let go of our identification with pain. It all happens in the present, and is gone…

But, again, who is suffering? We have not answered that question yet. We have only described the mechanics of suffering. When we are identified with our pain and are suffering, who is experiencing that? Is it our external sense of self? Our body/mind? Is it our awareness behind all of that? It gets to the heart of what self-inquiry is about. More importantly, it gets to the heart of what the witness is about, because without the witness there will be no relational self-inquiry. And without that, our sense of self will be externalized non-relationally in thoughts, feelings, the body, and our environment. That temporal condition of awareness will be where the suffering is.

Yet, is that who we are? Only if we are identified and habitually claim ourselves to be our external perceptions.

When we find our sense of self to be the witness, nothing will touch us there. We cannot suffer when we are *That*, no matter what the body and mind are doing. It is a fact that our consciousness does not suffer even when it is identified. It is only consciousness – that part of us that always has been. It does not change. Only the veneer of thoughts, feelings and materiality outside it changes. Inevitably, there is change in the external. But we never change inside, do we? Who then suffers?

The truth is that no one suffers, except those who are identified, and even that is an illusion – a belief in something that is temporary, a dream. Yet, it is very real to the one who is having the experience.

All of this is rather idyllic, and will mean little to us when we are in pain and identified with that experience. The same can be said of all who struggle with non-relational self-inquiry without sufficient presence of the witness. It is a tough slog. We do not intend to be insensitive about any of this. Whether we have the witness or not, we will feel compassion for all who suffer. Our humanity calls us instinctively to help others who are in need, and especially those who suffer.

The reason why spiritual teachers do what they do is because they want more than anything to aid everyone in moving beyond suffering into the unending peace and joy that is ever-present and available within us all.

There is only one condition that can save us from identification with the ups and downs of life. Only one condition that can save us from the struggles of the mind within itself. That is the witness, our inherent inner silence, which can be cultivated easily in daily deep meditation. Then true understanding becomes possible for us, and we find ourselves able to move beyond suffering, and wondering who was ever suffering.

The power of the witness with the clarity of self-inquiry playing upon it is a paradox and a mystery. Yet, more real than all we see in our external world of thoughts, feelings, and perceptions of the body and surrounding environment. The witness and relational self-inquiry are real because they make a tangible difference in the quality of our life. And what a difference it is!

Transcending Duality Through Divine Love

Speaking of paradox and mystery, as we find our sense of self residing ever more deeply in the stillness of our witness, in the shining transcendent glory of pure bliss consciousness, something inexplicable begins to happen. It contradicts what we may have been taught and come to believe about self-inquiry and the non-dual nature of existence. Yet, it cannot be denied.

Stillness moves of its own accord. It moves as an outward flow of divine love from within us.

As it does, the quality of stillness is retained. We find that our life has become a never-ending expression of stillness in action. Our natural ability to allow what is happening in life to play on the screen of our silent witness, remaining unidentified with the drama, leads to a dynamic in awareness we could not imagine before. We find ourselves engaged in doing many things, without doing anything. We have no pressing desires. Yet, desire is functioning. We see suffering and move to relieve it. We see need and move to fill it. We see beauty and move to honor it. Life becomes a dance. All the world becomes our sacred temple, and we move naturally in *That*, without moving at all. We are moved by divine love and by *That* alone. And there is no moving at all in that situation. It is *stillness in action*.

In this outpouring of divine love there is eternal stillness, and an ongoing transcendence of duality. This is what life is in the non-duality that is described in vedanta and yoga.

Some have claimed that this is the end of the ego. Well, maybe by someone's definition it is, but it is certainly not the end person. Rather it is the expansion of the person to the level of divine expression. It is correct to say that enlightenment is the end of identification and the simultaneous expansion of divine engagement. It is the ultimate example of less becoming more.

Even as we claim no part in the world, we will be very active in it. For this is the nature of pure consciousness and the enlightenment it yields – the constant expansion of stillness in this transparent existence, exploding it from the inside with love and goodness.

It is nothing new. It has been going on all the time, you know. In our realization, we are only coming on board consciously with a process that was always there and is eternal. We were only out of step for a short time while we were identified with the drama of life, created like a dream within us. When we find ourselves to be the *One* behind it all, we see it for what it is – a process that always was and always will be. Our eternal nothingness becoming everything we have imagined in a constant outpouring of divine love.

A Confirmation of Unity

Believing in the true nature of existence has value. It can inspire us to undertake the means for realizing that truth. This is why it is beneficial to study, at least until we see the truth manifesting directly within ourselves. Then we will know its attributes by our own experience, as seen from within our witness which is beyond all experience.

On the other hand, if we have never studied a high philosophical ideal representing the true nature of existence, if we begin a simple and effective practice like deep meditation for any reason at all – for health, for happiness, for more success in life – the result will be the same. Ultimately, our spiritual realization is not about what we believe. It is about what we become, and that is about the gradual purification and opening of our inner neurobiology. This is human spiritual transformation.

Having said that, we also know that the mind will come along. As the grip of the habit of identification with our thoughts, feelings and perceptions is loosened, so too will the external expression of these aspects of our nature become more peaceful and radiant. Then we are able to inquire about the true nature of our life and all of existence without a lot of mental struggles. This condition of peaceful radiance has sometimes been referred to as having a shining quality.

Paradoxically, it is this shining radiance, the movement of inner silence outward from within us, that brings us surely into a direct realization of the non-dual nature of existence. This is rarely discussed in considering a pure path of self-inquiry. Why? Because, pure vedantic self-inquiry may mechanically discard the existence of anything outside the void of awareness. Even awareness itself is released, because, we cannot know it without a sense of *"I,"* and there can be no sense of *"I"* if there is nothing that exists to comprehend it.

Nevertheless, here we are.

If we honor the appearance of our present perceptions, and the fact that we are behind and within these as the silent inner witness, then, in time, we will come to know that the realization of non-duality is the merging of these two. Enlightenment is the merging of energy with awareness.

This little-discussed later stage, where stillness becomes radiant and active, results in all of our activities and experiences being penetrated/illuminated by moving stillness – shining, as it were. And we become very attracted to residing in *That*, for we know instinctively that it is our *Self*.

This is the true realization of non-duality, which is a unification, rather than a separation of undifferentiated consciousness from the rest of life. Even as we reside in stillness, we will be active, and the qualities of the divine will be expressing in that way.

This is a confirmation of unity, and it will be seen by us and by everyone who is around us. Unity is the outpouring of divine love in every day activity. It is not the appearance of it (behaving in a particular way), but the internal fact of it, which cannot be mimicked for long. No matter what anyone has ever said about enlightenment, what it is or what it is not, we can only know it in experience as an expression of our own inner silence, which to us will not seem like an expression at all. It is an abiding, because we are forever at one with absolute stillness. And in this abiding, we are far more dynamic than we ever were before we came to rest in our own *Self*.

It has been said that final enlightenment requires a confirmation on the level of the mind. Perhaps it is so. In the end, that is why we have self-inquiry, so the mind may release and allow what already is. Allow us to be what we have always been – eternal divine love. After the neurobiological transformation and the emergence of outpouring divine love, it will be the intellect which finally reaches the point of saying, *Ahhh* ... and release.

Then we will be beyond relying on external philosophies or teachings. We will be describing unity in our own words.

By applying all available means in a balanced way, and by inquiring, we come to know the truth of the witness within, and the confirmation of unity will not be far behind. We will find mind and the world dancing with joy on the surface of our infinite ocean of being.

We are *That*...

Further Reading and Support

Yogani is an American spiritual scientist who, for more than thirty years, has been integrating ancient techniques from around the world which cultivate human spiritual transformation. The approach he has developed is non-sectarian, and open to all. In the order published, his books include:

Advanced Yoga Practices – Easy Lessons for Ecstatic Living
A large user-friendly textbook providing 240 detailed lessons on the AYP integrated system of yoga practices.

The Secrets of Wilder – A Novel
The story of young Americans discovering and utilizing actual secret practices leading to human spiritual transformation.

The AYP Enlightenment Series
Easy-to-read instruction books on yoga practices, including:

- *Deep Meditation – Pathway to Personal Freedom*
- *Spinal Breathing Pranayama – Journey to Inner Space*
- *Tantra – Discovering the Power of Pre-Orgasmic Sex*
- *Asanas, Mudras and Bandhas – Awakening Ecstatic Kundalini*
- *Samyama – Cultivating Stillness in Action, Siddhis and Miracles*
- *Diet, Shatkarmas and Amaroli – Yogic Nutrition and Cleansing for Health and Spirit*
- *Self Inquiry – Dawn of the Witness and the End of Suffering*
- *Bhakti and Karma Yoga – The Science of Devotion and Liberation Through Action*
- *Eight Limbs of Yoga – The Structure and Pacing of Self-Directed Spiritual Practice*

For up-to-date information on the writings of Yogani, and for the free *AYP Support Forums*, please visit:

www.advancedyogapractices.com

CPSIA information can be obtained at www.ICGtesting.com
Printed in the USA
LVOW101820200113

316455LV00022B/1218/A